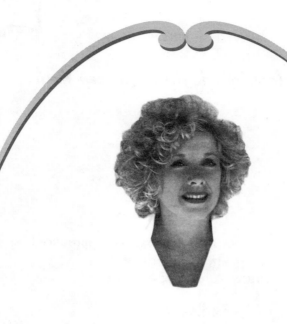

Weight Loss

&

Cellulite Control

The Healthy Healing Library Series

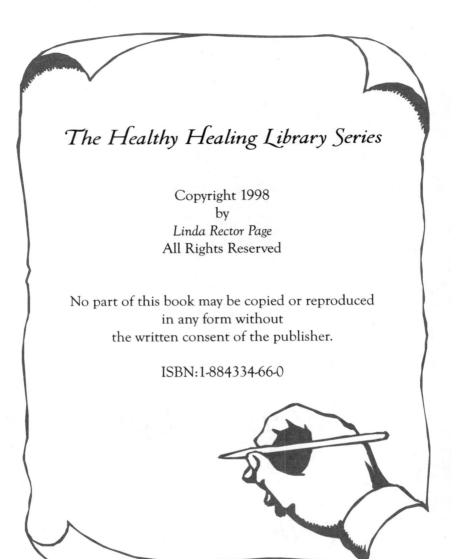

Published by Healthy Healing Publications, 1998
P.O. 436, Carmel Valley, CA 93924

About the Author....

L inda Page has been working in the
fields of nutrition and herbal medicine
both professionally and as a personal lifestyle choice, since the early seventies. She is
a certified Doctor of Naturopathy and Ph.D., with extensive experience in formu-
lating herbal combinations. She received a Doctor of Naturopathy from the Clayton
College of Natural Health in 1988, and a Ph.D. in Nutritional Therapy from the
American Holistic College of Nutrition in 1989. She is a member of both American and California Naturopathic Medical Associations.

Linda opened and operated the *"Rainbow Kitchen,"* a natural foods restaurant,
then became a working partner in The Country Store Natural Foods store. She is
the founder and formulator of *Crystal Star Herbal Nutrition,* a manufacturer of
over 250 premier herbal compounds, carried in natural food stores in the U.S.
and around the world.

Linda has written four books and a Library Series of specialty books in the
field of natural healing. Today, she is the editor-in-chief of a national monthly,
natural health newsletter, *The Natural Healing Report.* She has a weekly CBS News
TV segment where she discusses a wide range of natural healing topics, and she
has her own weekly, one-hour radio talk show program called "The World of
Healthy Healing." Linda also lectures around the country, contributes articles to
national publications, is regularly featured on radio and television, and is an ad-
junct professor at Clayton College of Natural Health.

Continuous research in all aspects of the alternative healing world has been
the cornerstone of success for her reference work *Healthy Healing* now in its tenth
edition, with sales of almost a million books.

Cooking For Healthy Healing, now in its second revised edition, is a companion
to *Healthy Healing.* It draws on both the recipes from the Rainbow Kitchen and
the more defined, lifestyle diets that she has developed for healing. *Cooking For
Healthy Healing* contains 33 diet programs, and over 900 healthy recipes.

In *How To be Your Own Herbal Pharmacist,* Linda addresses the rising appeal of
herbs and herbal healing in America. This book is designed for those wishing to
take more definitive responsibility for their health through individually developed herbal combinations.

Linda's party reference book, *Party Lights,* written with restaurateur and chef
Doug Vanderberg, takes healthy cooking one step further by adding fun to a good
diet.

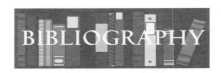

BIBLIOGRAPHY

"Does Getting Older Mean Getting Heavier." *Delicious!* Feb. 1998

Marcusen, Charlyn, Ph.D. "Weight Management- Skills for your Health." *Women's Health Journal.* May/June 1997

"The New Science of Perfect Eating." *First for Women.* 9/29/97

Leek, Richard, Ph.D. "Olestra? Just Say No!" *The ANMA & AANC Journal.* Feb & March 1996.

Berger, Laurie. "The Lowdown on Natural Fat Fighters." *Vegetarian Times.* January 1998

Gittleman, Ann L. "The New Diet Equation." *Let's Live.* Jan. 1997

Straus, Karen. "The Vegetarian Zone." *Vegetarian Times.* Jan 1997

Fraser, Laura. "The Latest Diet Drug." *Glamour.* March 1998

Mowrey, Daniel, Ph.D. *Fat Management! The Thermogenic Factor.* Victory Pub. © 1994

King, Jos. "The Secret to Weight Loss." *Whole Foods.* March 1998

"What Does The American Public Eat." *Delicious!* Nov. 1996

"The Good and the Bad of Fats and Oils." *Whole Foods.* Sept. 1997

"Pyruvate: Energy Metabolite Increases Endurance, Burns Fat and Supports Weight Loss." *Nutrition News.* Vol XX1, no.9

Blass, Donna. "Lose Weight, Inches & Cellulite With Our Customized Herbal Cures." *First for Women.* 2/2/98

Sears, Barry, PhD. *Mastering The Zone.* Harper Collins Inc. ©1997

"Fat-free and Fatter." *Men's Health.* May 1997

"Health Report." *Time.* December 1997

Books In The Library Series

※ *Renewing Female Balance*
※ *Sexuality - Enhancing Your Body Chemistry*
※ *Do You Have Blood Sugar Blues?- coming soon!*
※ *A Fighting Chance For Weight Loss & Cellulite Control*
※ *The Energy Crunch & You*
※ *Gland & Organ Health - coming soon!*
※ *Heart & Circulation - coming soon!*
※ *Detoxification & Body Cleansing to Fight Disease*
※ *Allergy Control & Management; Fighting Asthma*
※ *Ageless Vitality - Revealing the Secrets of Anti-Aging*
※ *Stress Management, Depression & Addictions*
※ *Colds & Flu & You - Building Optimum Immunity*
※ *Fighting Infections with Herbs - Controlling STDs*
※ *Beautiful Skin, Hair & Nails Naturally- coming soon!*
※ *Don't Let Your Food Go to Waste - coming soon!*
※ *Do You Want to Have a Baby? Natural Prenatal Care*
※ *Menopause & Osteoporosis - Taking Charge*
※ *Boosting Immunity With Power Plants*
※ *Herbal Therapy For Kids- coming soon!*
※ *Renewing Male Health & Energy*
※ *Cancer - Can Alternative Therapies Really Help?*
※ *Fatigue Syndromes - CFS, Candida, Lupus, Fibromyalgia*
※ *Overcoming Arthritis - coming soon!*

Dr. Page's written papers are thoroughly researched - through empirical observation as well as from documented evidence. Studies are ongoing and updated at Healthy Healing Publications, P.O. Box 436, Carmel Valley, CA 93924.

As affordable, high quality health
care in America becomes more difficult to
finance and obtain, natural therapies and personal
wellness techniques are receiving more attention and favor. Over
75% of Americans now use some form of natural health care,
from vitamins, to cleansing diets, to guided imagery, to herbal
supplements.

Everyone needs more information about these methods to
make informed health care choices for themselves and their fami-
lies. The Healthy Healing Library Series was created to answer
this need - with inexpensive, up-to-date books on the subjects
people want to hear about the most.

The lifestyle therapy programs discussed in each book have
been developed over the last fifteen years from the responses
and successful healing results experienced by literally thousands
of people. In addition, the full time research team at Healthy
Healing Publications, Inc. investigates herbs, herbal combinations and herbal therapies from around the world for their avail-
ability and efficacy. You can feel every confidence that the rec-
ommendations are synthesized from real people with real problems who got real results.

Herbal medicines are highlighted in these books because
they are in the forefront of science today. Herbal healing has
the proven value of ancient wisdom and a safety record of centuries. Science can only quantify, isolate, and assay to under-
stand. Herbs respond to these methods, but they are so much
more than the sum of their parts. God shows his face to us in
herbs. They, too, have an ineffable quality.

Fortunately for us, our bodies know how to
use herbs without our brains having
to know why.

Table of Contents

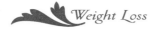

Weight Loss

*This small book can make a big difference
in your diet program.*

There's no doubt about it. Study after study shows it. It's getting harder to control our weight in America.

Some of the latest statistics are almost beyond belief:

Weight loss is a national obsession in America. Yet health experts say the U.S. is in an "obesity explosion." **A frightening 33% (about 65 million) adults in the United States are obese.**

Almost everybody is eating less fat. Most of us are exercising at least once a week. Yet another 58 million U.S. adults are overweight.

This doesn't count kids, who are rapidly becoming an overweight generation. A new study from *The New England Journal of Medicine*, shows that the probability that obese children over the age of 6 will become obese adults now exceeds 50%, compared to less than 10% for non-obese children. (This is certainly an added incentive for parents *and* kids to get weight under control at an early age.)

At any given time, over 25 million Americans are seriously dieting. **More than 50% of women, 44% of high school girls and 25% of men are trying to lose weight right now.** Most are struggling.

Regardless of our intentions, we eat a lot of fried, fatty, microwaved foods. Americans eat 31% more fat than they did in 1900. The telecommunications age has radically reduced the demand for physical labor. Americans expend 75% fewer exercise calories than they did in 1900. **Obesity has grown between 500 and 800% since the beginning of the 20th century.**

Today, everyone knows that obesity sets the stage for health problems all through life. High cholesterol and coronary artery disease (still the number one killer of adults) are just two of the problems linked to obesity. Last year, 300,000 deaths in the U.S. resulted from obesity-related diseases. Some studies show that being grossly overweight is now the second-leading cause of death in America, after smoking-related illnesses.

The financial burden is enormous. Health care costs to tax-payers, insurers and medical services due to obesity are $70 billion a year. This doesn't even count the $33 billion we spend annually on weight control products and services.

We're all desperately trying, but obviously, the answers to weight control aren't simple. That's because dieting alone isn't the whole answer. Exercise alone isn't the answer. Will power isn't even the answer. (I'll explain why later in this book.) Most serious dieters are able to lose about 10% of their body weight on a strict diet. Yet, 95% of all dieters gain back all the weight they lost within 5 years. Sometimes dieting can actually lead to additional weight gain.

Even drastic diets don't make much of a difference in the long run. Most people who repeatedly diet and fail, follow a "crash and burn" philosophy.... crash dieting to burn calories fast, without any real change in lifestyle or eating habits. Crash diets, especially those that are almost totally fat-free, are impossible to stick with, intolerable for a normal lifestyle, and even dangerous to health because they are so unbalanced. (Crash dieting also leads to the development of eating disorders in some people.) In the end, crash dieters get burned by gaining the weight back.

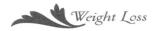

Weight control today has to be a strategy of prevention lifestyle - an attitude of achieving what I call a *balanced body*; one that is nourished, full of energy and at a comfortable, realistic body weight.

Common sense is still the best approach for permanent weight loss. Even though Americans will probably never stop looking for the *miracle magic bullet* for slimness, everyone is slowly realizing that good nutrition has to be front and center for permanent results.

Weight control is part of a sound nutritious eating plan, rather than a struggle with the latest diet fad. Weight problems are largely a result of imbalances in the body created by imbalances in diet and lifestyle. Natural therapies work primarily by rebalancing your body to create homeostasis (a stable state of equilibrium). People are also becoming more motivated for health reasons to lose weight. They are looking for weight control solutions that will last a lifetime and are willing to make the necessary lifestyle changes to do it.

Here are factors, besides diet, that affect your weight control:
- **Glandular activity.** Glandular substances like adrenaline, insulin, and thyroid hormones are very sensitive to nutritional deficiencies, environmental pollutants, chemicalized foods, and man-made hormones. Any or all of these can lead to impaired thyroid activity and unbalanced insulin levels, which adversely affect calorie-burning activity.

The glands are tied to seasonal rhythms, too. If you add a few pounds every fall and winter, you are validating the fact that our bodies are still influenced by the bio-rhythms from the ancient days of our species. When cold weather arrives, we put on a few pounds to prepare for winter.

• **Hypothyroidism.** Since WWII, an above average number of people have thyroid problems; many experts think this is the result of the incredible number of chemicals and environmental pollutants and hormones that have entered our society since the war and put a strain on glandular health. Over 25,000 new chemicals become part of our culture every year. And today, hypothyroidism is a common problem. A poorly functioning thyroid results in sluggish metabolism. When your metabolism is low, you use food less efficiently and you tend to eat more to make up for low energy. Most people with underactive thyroids (hypothyroidism) have a weight problem. Foods like caffeine, sugar, and alcohol can exhaust your thyroid and lead to low metabolism.

• **Sluggish liver.** Environmental pollutants and food chemicals affect more than your glands. They keep all body processes from flowing freely. Of the 4.5 billion pounds of pesticides we dump yearly in the U.S, over 77% are used in agricultural sectors to produce your food! Their toxic build-up can cause an overload on the organs responsible for detoxification, like the liver and the kidneys. **The liver is also the chief organ for fat digestion,** for excreting excess fats like cholesterol, and for regulating fat-involved hormones like estrogen. An exhausted liver can be the reason for unexplained weight gain and poor elimination. All body systems slow down, especially fat metabolism and digestion when the liver is sluggish.

• **Brain chemistry.** Can the chemicals in the brain really affect weight control? People who just can't seem to shake food cravings may have brain chemistry to blame.

Experiences which bring pleasure trigger the release of dopamine, a chemical in the brain which scientists believe con-

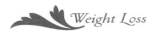
trols addictions. When you are exposed to the trigger experience again, like eating a candy bar, directly or indirectly (somebody else could be eating it), dopamine floods your brain synapses and your cravings get stronger. Fava beans are a natural rich source of dopamine which may help curb cravings.

Other experts feel the brain chemical serotonin is the missing link. Serotonin increases the feel-good side of dopamine, as well as norepinephrine which increases alertness and energy. Serotonin is also thought to decrease appetite by reducing stress-related overeating, increasing the feeling of fullness and enhancing general well-being.

Remember fen/phen? This once very popular diet-drug combo worked by altering brain chemistry to control appetite.

Weight loss drugs like fen/phen and Redux were developed to answer the brain's calling for food by modulating serotonin levels to decrease appetite. Americans thought they had finally found the "magic bullet" for weight loss. In 1996, the total number of prescriptions in the U.S. for fen/phen exceeded 18 million.

By 1997, the "bullet" had lost its magic. A substantial number of patients developed heart valve defects while on fen/phen. It was banned, leaving an enormous desire from the public for a safer alternative. *Meridia*, another serotonin-modulating drug, was approved as safer but clinical trials showed that it, too, has a downside. Almost ten percent of the subjects in one study had a significant rise in blood pressure. *Xenical*, a new weight loss drug that functions by blocking fat absorption in the gut, was expected to hit the shelves in autumn 1998. It has been delayed because of unpleasant side effects that increase as more fat is eaten, and links to breast cancer. *Xenical's* long term safety has not yet been established.

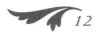

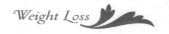

Is herbal phen/fen the answer?

Some people have turned to herb-based serotonin modulators (herbal phen/fen) as a safer way to fill the void of 18 million prescriptions left by fen/phen and Redux. As an herbalist who has worked with weight control problems for many years, I can tell you that some of the herbs in herbal phen/fen products can indeed help you lose weight when used properly.

Most herbal phen/fen combinations contain St. John's *wort*, *green tea, ephedra* and a variety of other natural diet aids. St. *John's wort*, although more often used by traditional herbalists as an anti-viral and anti-depressant, also works as an appetite suppressant through serotonin balancing activity in the brain. *Ephedra (ma huang)*, known for its bronchodilating effects, has a well-documented history of safety and effectiveness in weight loss combinations, as an appetite suppressant and thermogenic (fat burning) aid.

Is herbal phen/fen safe?

Many of the products work safely. A 1997 study done at the Obesity Research Center shows that a *St. John's wort/ephedra* combination can produce weight loss with minimal side effects. But use caution. Some manufacturers use synthetic or synthesized ephedrine, chemical cousin or drug derivative of the *ephedra* plant, and combine it with stimulants like caffeine in herbal phen/fen formulas. This type of concentrated isolate tends to be too harsh on the body, has a high potential for abuse and misuse and can cause side effects like heart palpitations.

I recommend using *ephedra* **only as a whole herb** in combination with other whole herbs like *green tea, kola nut, and St. John's wort* in an herbal fen/phen formula for the best weight loss results.

Unlike ephedrine, whole *ephedra* rarely causes side effects, especially in an herbal combination. (See pg. 65 for more information on *ephedra*) If you wish to avoid *ephedra*, look for a combination that contains *sida cordifolia*, a milder Ayurvedic herb with similar fat burning properties.

I have worked with herbal diet aids for years, and my office has a continuing natural product review process. Effective herbal phen/fen products include THERMO-CITRIN GINSENG™ by Crystal Star, PHENSOLUTION by Nature's Secret and ELIM/SLIM SUPREME by Gaia Herbs. Take the formulas only as directed and always make a balanced diet part of your weight management program.

What about " The Zone" diet? Is it right for you?

"The Zone" diet, developed by Barry Sears Ph.D., is very popular in the media today as people continually search for the perfect combination of foods that will help them lose weight easily. It is a 40-30-30 plan: 40% of calories come from carbohydrates, 30% come from protein (mostly from animal protein products), and 30% come from fat.

The diet is based on the premise that the dramatic increase in overweight Americans, (as well as heart disease and arthritis) is the result of carbohydrate overload. "Zone" researchers say that 75% of the U.S. population have a high insulin response to carbohydrates which causes them to get fat and stay fat, while the remaining 25% of us can eat as much pasta, refined carbohydrates (like white sugar and white flour), or even candy bars as we like and never gain any extra pounds. The name "Zone" refers to keeping the hormone insulin in a tight zone by eating specific ratios of carbohydrates to protein at each meal in order to achieve a state of hormonal balance that insures successful weight loss.

"Zone" advocates say that by lowering carbohydrate intake and limiting insulin production, your body will increase its production of *glucagon* which helps you burn fat. Some people say that the " Zone" diet is the only diet that has ever helped them to lose weight and keep it off. **But will it work for you?**

In my twenty-five years in the diet and health industry, I can tell you that variations on high protein diets have been around before. In the 70's, Dr. Richard Atkins promoted his famous Atkins diet which severely restricted carbohydrates and told Americans to "eat all the protein they wanted." The Atkins diet drove insulin levels too low, causing fatigue and irritability. The abnormally low ratio of carbohydrates to protein in this diet caused an over-acid, metabolic condition called ketosis.

In the 80's, many people, especially athletes, tried the Scarsdale diet, another high protein plan. I personally knew some of the athletes using the diet who found that the excessively high protein led to blood in their urine, a condition related to stress on the kidneys. I tried it myself, and did indeed lose weight, only to gain it back within a few months.

In my experience, high protein diets work only short term, possibly to boost healing or extra muscle development for athletes, but, invariably, with long term use the muscle turns into fat and kidney health suffers.

Of the new crop of diets advocating high protein, Dr. Sear's "Zone" diet is probably one of the safest. It does not completely restrict eating grains, nor does it suggest people eat as much protein as they want.

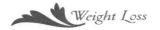

The real dangers are **"Zone clones,"** which do not restrict protein intake **at all**. Following one of those is not be a good idea. The true "Zone" diet developed by Sears, actually contains more carbohydrates than protein, and, therefore, is not considered harmful for the kidneys or ketogenic, causing acidosis or the presence of ketones in the blood or urine.

A big problem, in my opinion, with all the "zone" diets is that they focus on eating meat (albeit lean cuts) for their protein. "Zone diet" recipes use large amounts of red meat.

All the "Zone" diets recommend eating more protein than is advised in the daily U.S. RDA requirement of 63 grams for men over 25, and 50 grams for women over 25.

The average American already eats 80-120 grams of protein a day, and there's no question that we consume fat at record levels. Rich meats, cheeses, and butter, once reserved for special occasions, are a routine part of the average diet.

Dr. Sears recommends 98 grams of protein daily for males and 77 grams for females. For many people, meat is hard to digest, and clogging up your elimination systems and arteries is not good for general health. People who do not eat red meat have a well-documented history of lower risk for heart disease, obesity, diabetes, osteoporosis and several types of cancer. They also play an important role in conserving water, topsoil and energy resources wasted by animal-based diets.

"Zone" diets fail to take advantage of vegetable protein sources vital to health, especially for vegetarians. Dr. Sears' diet makes a few suggestions for vegetarians who wish to "zone", but the protein in his diet still comes from meat. Many health experts feel that 30% of calories coming from animal protein is still too high and may lead to high cholesterol levels and heart disease.

Further, hormones and antibiotics are regularly injected into American meats and dairy products. We know that man-made estrogens can stack the deck against women by increasing their estrogen levels hundreds of times over normal levels.

Medical researchers are also realizing that women aren't the only ones endangered by the estrogen-imitating effects of these substances. Substantial new evidence shows that synthetic estrogens threaten male health with reproductive disorders, too. The most alarming statistics relate to sperm count and hormone driven cancers.

Zone supporters claim that carbohydrates are the culprit in our modern diet. Some Zone supporters believe that obesity, arthritis, heart attacks and even the shrinking of mankind is based on lack of adequate protein and too many carbohydrates in the diet. To some degree, especially in the case of refined carbohydrates like sugar and white flour, they may be right.

But I strongly disagree that health problems can be blamed on a diet rich in complex carbohydrates like whole grains. The reality is that most Americans actually eat too much protein and too much fat, and **not enough** complex carbohydrates from whole grains, fruits and vegetables. I have been developing healing diets for many years for real people with real problems. Dense grains, like brown rice, barley, millet or wheat bran, pack a nutritional punch of valuable B vitamins, complex carbohydrates and minerals that everybody needs today.

Many people who eat a high carbohydrate diet, low in fat and protein, believe it is an effective way to lose weight and maintain a desirable size.

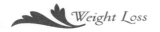

Entering A Healthier Zone

I, myself, have struggled with my weight all my life mostly as a result of a high stress lifestyle, a junk food diet and the use of the Pill (which in its early versions had very high levels of estrogen). Today, as a much thinner person, I find that a well-balanced diet that helps me feel good and maintain my weight is based on fresh, whole, enzyme-rich foods. The majority of my meals consist of complex carbohydrates from dense grains like brown rice, beans, peas, and plenty of fruits and vegetables. I eat a green salad every day, and most of my protein comes from the sea. The little fat I do eat comes from EFA's in seafoods and sea vegetables. I never recommend a no-fat diet for anyone. Fat helps to slow down the rate at which carbohydrates enter the bloodstream, thus decreasing insulin and fat storage. I find that a largely vegetarian, natural foods diet works best for me.

A "Veggie & Seafood Zone diet" may be a healthier alternative to the high meat Zone diet, especially if you need a little more protein in your life to balance out your sugar cravings.

Chronic stress or diabetes cause protein needs to increase, so protein is a valuable tool for normalizing. There are complete proteins available in the vegetable kingdom, and fish is a healthier alternative to beef, pork or poultry (all routinely injected with hormone disrupting chemicals). If you want to get a little extra protein in your diet, include some of the following healthy protein foods: all legumes, soy foods, blue-green algae, spirulina, chlorella, brewer's yeast, wheat germ, nuts, seeds, dark green leafy vegetables like kale and chard and cruciferous vegetables like broccoli and cauliflower. Although, Dr. Sears suggests that many of these foods are at an unbalanced ratios of carbohydrates to proteins, I can tell you that I've been eating them for years and I've lost weight and kept it off.

Vegetable proteins work synergistically in a process called *protein complementarity*, like the vegetable protein combos below:

• Stew or soup from legumes and whole wheat flat bread- for a balanced meal, rich in protein, carbohydrates and fiber.

• Black beans and rice- for an optimum source of absorbable protein that can even alkalize an over-acid body.

• Sprouts of all kinds are an excellent source of natural, cleansing protein which provides vitamin A, B-complex, C, D, and E, and enzymes, essential fatty acids and minerals.

Why doesn't will power work? Essentially, it's because the human body is made to be a self-balancing, and largely, self-healing mechanism. When your body becomes unbalanced, because of illness or pollutants or dieting, it will try to rebalance and right itself when the illness or diet are over. It does this by **cravings** (communications from your body to you that ask you for different nutrients in certain foods). For example, if you are deficient in B vitamins, you might crave brown rice.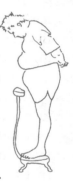

Is willpower necessary? Not really. Balance through a variety of nutrient-rich foods, and moderation is really the key. You can see that in the craving mechanism, which affects almost everybody after a fad or Zone-type diet, the more will power you have, the more you may be actually *imbalancing* your body.... even to the point of harming yourself. (People with eating disorders often have an enormous amount of will power.)

Can decadent-tasting food ever be healthy? People have been asking themselves this ever since the Puritan era.

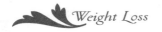

Modern dieters have been struggling with answers since the seventies. In the nineties, it is virtually a national hysteria.

If it tastes incredibly yummy, should we be eating it? The "food police" warn us away from yet another food or cuisine almost every week. With the best of intentions, all sorts of health professionals bombard us daily with the need to keep our diets totally fat-free. Market forces respond, and we reduce calories, fat, sugar and salt in everything we can get our hands on. It's the best way to eat, right?

Maybe not, if it's at the expense of eating whole, live foods.

Today's fat-free effort stems from the fact that the Standard American Diet is so regularly loaded with saturated fats. And the typical American way of dealing with a problem is to take drastic steps all at once.

In the case of weight loss, as with most health problems, it just doesn't work. Even with all the low-fat and fat-free foods available, Americans still consume almost 33% of their calories from fat. Even the most conservative medical thinking states that for cardiovascular health we should be eating only 25 to 30% of our calories as fat.

For weight control, especially as we age, fat should be about 20% or less of daily food intake. This means that most Americans still need to reduce their fat intake by **13% or more.**

Are the new fat-free, calorie-free "designer" foods healthy? Most designer foods, made from fat-free, sugar-free, salt-free, calorie-free chemical substances, offer minimal nutrition. Some offer no nutrients at all. **I call these foods, "non-foods."** The nutrition label reads zero. And that's what your body gets from the product ...nothing.

We need to use a little common sense here. The reason our bodies need food is for nourishment, sustenance.... life. Designer non-foods may be useful as a snack for a short dieting period for someone who constantly overeats. They fool the body into feeling satisfied, but we shouldn't kid ourselves that they are foods or provide nutrition.

Fake fats especially fool your tastebuds, not your stomach. One new study revealed that people who replaced 20% of their fat intake with fat substitutes, such as Olestra, (found in many fat free potato chips), were still hungry at the end of the day and they had eaten twice as much food as normal!

Real fats slow down digestion - fat substitutes don't. Some, like Olestra, actually speed up digestion and can cause griping pains or diarrhea.

Olestra has also been found to prevent the absorption of certain nutrients vital to health, such as vitamin A, D, E, K (necessary for blood-clotting) and beta carotene. In one study, eating 16 Olestra potato chips for 8 weeks reduced blood carotene levels by 50%! Carotenes are some of the best cancer fighting nutrients available. In animal studies, Olestra was linked to liver-cell damage and potential cancer risk. We still do not know its long term effects on humans.

By targeting your weight loss diet for "no fat," you open up your body to health risks. **It's back to the craving mechanism again (pg. 19). If you try to eliminate all the fat from your diet, you end craving fatty foods.**

Unfortunately, the advertising of fat-free foods, especially snacks and sweets, implies that we can eat as much as we want of them and not put on weight. But people tend to feel like they're getting a free ride and eat too much. Or, they compensate by eating sugary foods to fill the hole left by eliminating fat. Don't forget that many fat-free foods still have plenty of calories.

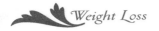

Watch out for items with claims like "98% Fat Free." These foods are only 98% fat free by **weight**. The significant number is the percentage of calories from **fat**. For example, whole milk is only 4% fat by weight, but 50 % of its calories come from fat. Further, many products that claim to be "lite" can be very deceiving. Lite mayo is still more than 75% fat!

Do you like a food well enough to wear it? How do so-called "forbidden foods," like fat, salt, sugar and caffeine fit into the weight control picture?

For instance, what role does fat play in your body's health? Fat isn't all bad. It's our body's chief source of energy, and essential for synthesizing essential fatty acids in small amounts. A small amount of fat provides energy, warmth and membrane health. **I never recommend a no-fat diet for anyone.** Fat plays a part in hormone, gland and prostaglandin functions, too. Mono-unsaturated fats, like olive oil, are definitely healthy for liver metabolism and cholesterol balance.

In fact, you can fight fat with fat. Not all fats make people fat. Omega-3 fatty acids actually increase metabolic rate. They rid the body of excess fluids and help heighten energy levels. The best sources of omega-3 fatty acids are flaxseed oil and cold water fish like salmon.

Essential fatty acids, EFAs, are not produced by the body and need to be synthesized from fats in the diet. They help cells work, keep organs from deteriorating prematurely, provide moisture and softness to skin, vagina, and bladder, and boost brain activity. An EFA deficiency actually increases appetite, promotes obesity, high cholesterol and hypertension. After water, protein and carbohydrates, essential fatty acids are needed by the body more than any other nutrient. The gray matter of the brain alone is 50% EFA's! **For vegetarians, I recommend adding 1 to 2 TBS. of flax seed or grapeseed oil to your salad dressing for therapeutic EFA's.**

Gamma linolenic acid, or GLA, is a fatty acid essential to healthy metabolism. Sources of GLA are borage seed oil, black currant oil and EVENING PRIMROSE oil, which I recommend for women for PMS and especially during menopause when estrogen levels decrease.

Yet weight loss seems to be our only operative reason, so we try to avoid all fats all the time. This causes constant hunger - the delicate balance between fat storage and fat utilization is upset, and the body's ability to use fat for energy is reduced. Eating fatty, fried, or junk foods particularly aggravates this imbalance. The person winds up with "empty calories" and more cravings. Since calories from fat do not cause a person to feel full, many people continue to eat fatty foods way past a healthy limit.

But what about the bad fats? What fats should we avoid?

You only need about **5%** of the calories you consume to come from fat in order to produce enough essential fatty acids for good health.

Fats are not metabolized right away. They're often stored in adipose tissue which has an almost unlimited capacity to contain them. Fat becomes non-moving energy in these storage depots, and a ready storehouse for body toxins and environmental pollutants that would be eliminated under normal body conditions.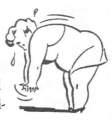

Fat-related diseases go way beyond obesity. Atherosclerosis, the cause of most heart disease and strokes, is directly linked to excess dietary fat and plaque rupture. A fatty, meat-based diet is related to some cancers, notably breast and colon cancer. A 1996 study of 422 women in Uruguay shows a 4.2 times greater risk for breast cancer in women who consume large amounts of red meat. *Note: The most significant risk for breast cancer is associated with eating fried meat. Fried or barbecued meats contain a significantly higher content of carcinogens than broiled meats.* Beware!

Here are the fats to limit in your diet:
• **Saturated fats,** found chiefly in red meats, cheeses and butter are the main culprits in most degenerative disease. Eating them regularly or to excess will almost certainly add pounds and can clog up your arteries. A little may be okay, a lot is not.

• **Trans fatty acids,** found in margarine, shortening products, and partially hydrogenated oils (in almost all potato chips), are not naturally occurring fats. They are produced when hydrogen atoms are added in the manufacturing process. Like saturated fats, they are very difficult for the body to process and use. They raise "bad" LDL cholesterol and lower "good" HDL cholesterol, decrease immune response and interfere with the body's natural process of detoxification. Trans fatty acids have also been linked to pregnancy and reproductive problems. They are the only fatty acid which has been found to raise lipoprotein, a risk factor for heart disease.

• **Refined oils,** like most supermarket oils, are treated with solvents, bleached, deodorized, and heated at high enough temperatures to destroy antioxidants and form free radicals. Look for oils that are extracted by an expeller or mechanical press.

Healthier choices for fats and oils to include in small quantities in your weight control diet: 1) monounsaturated fats, like canola or olive oil, are proven to actually lower blood cholesterol and ease constipation. 2) polyunsaturated fats, like flax seed or fish oils, are good sources of essential fatty acids.

Many women avoid salt as part of their weight loss diet so they won't retain excess fluid. Should we avoid all salt?

There is no denying that Americans consume too much salty restaurant food, salt-preserved animal products and salt-processed condiments. Whole industries have grown up around salt-free diet foods. Most people are aware today that too much salt can be a major factor in heart problems, high blood pressure and poor circulation. Our bodies retain extra fluid to compensate for too much salt.

Not so well known is the fact that excessive salt intake is involved in migraine headaches, aggressive, hyperactive behavior and poor gland function. Obviously a salt-free diet is good for someone who eats too much salt.

But no-salt can do just as much body harm as too much salt. Too little salt leads to fatigue, poor intestinal tone, stagnate blood, less mental acuity and nutrient transportation throughout the body. A recent *Lancet Journal* study of 11,000 people reveals that people who reported eating moderate amounts of salt were less likely to die from cardiovascular diseases.

A craving for salty foods may indicate that your body needs minerals. Sea vegetables, such as kelp, dulse or sushi nori provide these minerals and improve thyroid function and sluggish metabolism. Even if you have high blood pressure, once your body's salinity normalizes, you should bring back some natural salts like soy sauce, miso and herbal seasonings into your diet.

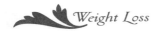

Is the bad rap on sugar too extreme?

The latest research shows that while most Americans are aware of the health problems and pitfalls of eating refined sugar, we as a nation are eating more sugar than ever. Some people say we are a nation addicted to sugar. The average person consumes 150 pounds of sugar per year.

Sugar offers quick energy, helps metabolism, and provides "closure" to digestive processes. **But most people don't know that sugar can actually suppress appetite, reducing the likelihood of overeating.** It's the reason we traditionally eat sweet things at the end of a meal.

However, regularly 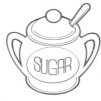 eating foods with large amounts of refined sugar causes abnormal insulin production in the body resulting in health problems like diabetes, hypoglycemia and obesity.

There is a strange dichotomy about sugar consumption in America today. Sugar restraint seems to be getting easier for very health conscious people who used to eat lots of sugar. Their diets now feature limited sweets, and their tastes have changed. For them, sweet things have returned to the places of honor they occupied in years past when sweet ingredients were hard to obtain. Except for fruits, these people see sweets as special treats, things to eat for celebrations, or tidbits of indulgence at the end of a party or a meal.

For others, especially people who try to live on fat-free diets, sugar has become a fat substitute for taste in their foods and they are eating more sugar than ever.

Then there's caffeine. It's America's favorite stimulant. Can it really help us control our weight? Lately, science has been giving us pause as we drink that morning cup of coffee. But is it as bad for us as the food police tell us?

Like most of mankind's other pleasures, there is good news and bad news about caffeine. We know it's a good appetite suppressant, and an effective, short term dieting aid. Most of us love that morning cup of coffee.

Caffeine has been hailed for centuries for its therapeutic benefits. Every major culture uses xanthine-containing plant stimulants like caffeine to overcome fatigue, handle pain, open breathing, control weight and increase circulation.

There is solid evidence for the positive effects of caffeine on mental performance, in terms of clearer thinking, shorter reaction time, and increased attention span. Caffeine expands alertness by releasing adrenaline into the bloodstream. It mobilizes circulatory fatty acids, facilitating greater energy production, sports endurance and work output. It benefits weight control by enhancing metabolism and fat burning (thermogenesis).

The carcinogenic effects often blamed on caffeine may be caused by the roasting process used in making coffee, tea and chocolate. Since *de-caffeinated* coffee is also implicated in some types of organ cancer, scientists are concluding that caffeine is not really the culprit - hydro-carbons produced from the roasting process are.

But too much caffeine from any source causes health problems like headaches and migraines, irritability and digestive upset. Excess caffeine produces oxalic acid in the system, causing health problems that could lead to disease.

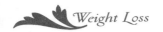

Caffeine also contributes to calcium loss through the urine increasing osteoporosis risk. As an addictive stimulant, it has drug-like side effects like jumpiness, mood swings, nervousness and heart palpitations. Caffeine leaches B vitamins, particularly thiamine, which controls stress. It can lodge in the liver restricting its proper function, and over time, it may constrict arterial blood flow. It is definitely involved in PMS symptoms, bladder infections, hypoglycemia and diabetic sugar reactions.

Preliminary studies reveal that chronic coffee drinkers have high blood homocysteine levels, a factor clearly related to heart disease and high cholesterol. Even drinking too much black tea may contribute to kidney stones in susceptible people.

Moderation is the key to caffeine use. Small amounts of caffeine *after* a meal can raise thermogenesis or calorie burning, and increase metabolic rate for weight loss. Over-use of caffeine exhausts the adrenals, and may cause hormonal imbalances to the point of becoming a factor in the growth of breast and uterine fibroids in women, and prostate trouble in men.

Caffeine may raise blood pressure so those with hypertension might avoid it altogether. It can lead to full-blown panic attacks in people with anxiety disorders. Pregnant women should also limit their consumption. More than 300mg per day of caffeine is linked to spontaneous abortion, intrauterine growth retardation and low birth weight.

Is there common sense in the food wilderness?

Human bodies are designed to assimilate a wide variety of foods. Our enzyme structure is capable of digesting thousands of diverse nutrients. Common sense, moderation and variety should be watchwords for a weight loss diet. It's really the same old story - a little is fine for health, a lot is not.

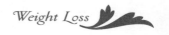
What's The Best Way To Get Started?

Changing diet composition is the passport to weight control. **If moderation is a key, then portion control is the password to moderation.** We've known this from the ancient Greeks to modern diet clinics. Why do we act differently? Probably because Americans like to take giant steps. Once we make a decision to act, we want to get out in front of a problem right away. That's not bad. It ain't what you do, it's the way that you do it.

The four keys to an effective weight control diet program are low fat, high fiber, regular exercise, and plenty of water. Add plenty of fresh vegetables. Have a green salad every day. Use only whole foods, light sweeteners, and low-fat ingredients.

There are almost as many different weight loss problems as there are people who have them.

I've identified six of the most common ones and developed comprehensive programs to address them. Each of the six plans has years of empirical success behind it. Once you make the big decision to be a thin person, analyze what your weight loss block really is.

Best results are achieved by working on the worst problem first. Identify your most prominent weight control problem, especially if there seems to be more than one.

As improvement is realized in the primary area, secondary problems are often overcome in the process. If lingering problem spots still exist, they may be addressed with additional supplementation after the first program is well underway and producing noticeable results.

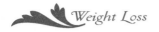

After identifying your personal difficulty, choose the weight loss options that most appeal to you. Follow directions carefully. Natural products work with your body to rebalance gland functions, so product activity is usually subtle and long-range for more permanent results.

Overdosing is generally not productive, nor will it increase effectiveness. Go slow, stick to it, improve your diet and your daily habits if necessary.

The goal is a balanced body at a healthy, realistic weight.

#1 Lazy metabolism and thyroid imbalance.

The thyroid gland produces hormones which profoundly influence the body's metabolic rate. A poorly functioning thyroid invariably results in sluggish metabolism. When your metabolism is low, you use food less efficiently and tend to eat more to make up for low energy. So most people with underactive thyroids, or hypothyroidism, have a weight problem. Since WWII an above average number of people have thyroid problems. Today, hypothyroidism is almost common, largely because of powerful environmental chemicals and pollutants that put such a strain on glandular health.

Factors that cause thyroid problems, decreasing the rate at which the body burns calories, include:

1) vitamin and mineral deficiencies, like potassium, iodine and B vitamins.

2) thyroid and pituitary exhaustion from over-stimulation by caffeine, sugar, and other stimulants.

3) substances that inhibit thyroid function, such as alcohol and thyroid-depressing drugs.

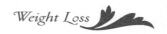

Check these body signs if you think your metabolism is low:
- lethargy and unusual fatigue (especially in the morning)
- swelling of the ankles, hands and eyelids
- chronic bloating, gas and indigestion after eating
- unusual depression and anxiety
- hair loss (especially in middle-aged women)
- unexplained obesity
- appearance of breast fibroids
- poor immune response

Natural solutions for a sluggish metabolism weight problem:
•Sea plants, rich in iodine and potassium, are a good choice to help regulate the body's metabolism and thyroid functions. A mineral-rich capsule combination with sea plants and metabolic stimulating herbs like Crystal Star's META-TABS™ helps balance the body while stimulating an active metabolic rate.

•A HOT SEAWEED bath with thyroid-stimulating ocean nutrients is also effective. Take a seaweed bath once a week along with a thermogenic combination of herbs that boost calorie-burning and increase long-range energy - like Crystal Star's THERMO-CITRIN GINSENG™ caps, ULTRA DIET PEP by Natural Balance, or DIET-PHEN by Source Naturals, an ephedra-free formula.

Note: Taking this type of compound with evening primrose oil as an essential fatty acid source boosts metabolism even more.

Other natural aids for normalizing metabolism include:
- **Chromium,** 200mcg to activate thermogenesis.
- **Carnitine,** about 250mg. with CoQ_{10}, 60mg daily.
- **Tyrosine,** 500mg for hypothyroidism.
- **Fat digesting enzymes,** like Prevail FAT ENZYME.

Diet tips for lazy metabolism and thyroid imbalance:

• Add 2 tablespoons of chopped, dried sea vegetables from an Oriental market or health food store to your daily diet (or have six pieces of sushi) to recharge your thyroid.

• Thermogenic spices like cinnamon, cayenne, mustard and ginger to your diet speed up your fat burning process. Try dipping raw veggies in mustard throughout the day. One teasp. of mustard can increase metabolism 25% for up to 3 hours!

#2 Overeating and eating too much fat and calories.

Overeating on empty calories (like junk food), is the downfall of most dieters. Overeaters usually diet by eating one large meal a day and then try to eat nothing the rest of the time. That single meal often contains more calories than three or four smaller meals!

Eating only once a day is a diet that's almost impossible to maintain because of society's conventions. Gnawing hunger for long periods makes the dieter irritable and miserable. So the dieter not only gains weight but also loses a positive outlook and peace of mind. This type of diet taxes willpower to the max and makes the dieter want to binge to compensate for the torture.

Overeating is often the result of poor food choices. Our body expects us to give it nutrients to work with - for energy and to feel satisfied. If you're not getting a balanced diet from whole grains and fresh vegetables, your body may keep calling for more food for energy and you'll overeat. If you're giving your body non-food foods like chemical-laced foods or microwaved foods that kill the food enzymes, your body won't recognize any nutrition, so you'll keep feeling hungry and you may overeat.

Overeating is aggravated in America by our lifestyle habits. Americans spend 45% of every food dollar on eating out, and restaurant portion sizes keep getting bigger as Americans demand more food for their money.

A Reminder About Fat

Fat is still the body's chief source of energy. Fat contains a higher number of calories and heat energy per gram of weight than either protein or carbohydrates. In fact, our bodies naturally convert unused carbohydrates and proteins into fat in order to store them as a source of energy.

You must have a certain amount of good fat in the bloodstream for health. So a person who does away with every bit of fat is usually tired, frequently malnourished, has chronic indigestion, and is constantly hungry. The average overweight person often has too high blood sugar and too low fat levels.

Nevertheless, the importance of cutting back on fat cannot be overstated. You can eat two to three times more volume of low-fat foods than high fat foods, and still lose weight. I feel a healthy body is the real target for weight control, because a healthy body is balanced and doesn't tend to accumulate fat.

Signs that you may have an overeating problem:
• you binge on junk foods, especially fatty and sugary foods, about every ten days.
• you eat all your calories at one meal and try to eat nothing for the rest of the day when you're dieting. (Most people can't do it.)
• you have second and third helpings at a meal but still feel hungry.

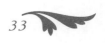

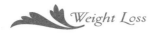

Natural solutions for an overeating weight problem:

• Use super green supplement foods to help control your appetite if you binge on fatty foods. Green foods like alfalfa, spirulina, chlorella and barley grass between meals can almost instantly decrease cravings for high-calorie foods and they offer a green energy lift that can carry throughout your day.

Green superfoods increase oxygen efficiency, and raise metabolic and energy levels. The protein in green superfoods may increase metabolism 30%, compared to only a 10% increase in a carbohydrate-based meal. Green foods also decrease the fatigue experienced after a low-protein meal.

Consider having a green superfood drink, like Crystal Star's ENERGY GREEN™ in the middle of the afternoon. (I like it mixed with apple juice.) You'll find green drinks at your local health food store and most juice bars carry them to add to your smoothies. You can get an extra energy lift from amino acids. Crystal Star's AMINO ZYME™ caps has aminos especially helpful for weight loss as well as enzymes to assimilate them properly.

• Try an herbal appetite control supplement, like Crystal Star's APPE-TIGHT™ caps with St. John's wort, if overeating is your diet problem. A combination like this works even better when taken with sea vegetables like kelp or dulse (from Maine Coast Sea Vegetables), or a good metabolism-stimulating compound, like Crystal Star META-TABS™ with sea vegetables.

Other natural weight control solutions for overeaters:
• **Chromium,** 200mcg to activate thermogenesis.
• **Phenylalanine and Carnitine,** to suppress appetite.
• **Bromelain** 1500mg daily for increased metabolism of fats.

• **Water** - can help an overeater get past weight loss plateaus. Drink it, and all liquids before eating, to suppress appetite and maintain a high metabolic rate.

• **Pyruvate**, a pyruvic acid salt, can help you lose excess fat. Pyruvic acid is a metabolite which aids in the transformation of blood sugar into energy. A study done at the Pittsburgh School of Medicine shows that taking pyruvate, along with a 1000 calorie a day liquid diet, increases weight loss 37% and fat loss 50% for obese women when compared to those on a low-fat diet alone. Red apples are a rich source of pyruvate, but to effectively stimulate weight loss, researchers recommend 5 grams of supplemental pyruvate daily.

Note: *Pyruvate is associated with some adverse effects, such as occasional gas, bloating, and diarrhea.* One expert reports that taking 30 grams of pyruvate bound to calcium or sodium (the only two forms available), can make you feel pretty bad.

• **Chitosan**, derived from a component of the exoskeletons of shellfish, is a natural product that reduces absorption of dietary fats and cholesterol in the intestines. Chitosan is an indigestible fiber that attaches to fat in the stomach before it is metabolized, then carries the fat (and cholesterol) through normal body channels to be eliminated instead of absorbed. A Japanese study compared chitosan to 22 different fiber foods and found that it was a stronger fat magnet than any other fiber, cutting the fat assimilated by almost half as much as a control group. A 1994 report shows that test subjects lost 8% of body weight in four weeks with chitosan.

Note: *Although there are reports that chitosan has been used for over 2 decades without side effects, some experts note that along with helping to block the absorption of fat in the gut, chitosan also interferes with the absorption of some minerals and fat-soluble vitamins. As with pyruvate, gastrointestinal problems may result.*

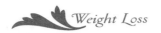

Diet tips for overeating and eating too much fat and calories:

• Control your portions. Even if you eat the right kinds of foods, eating them to excess will keep your stomach stretched.

• Eat more nutritious foods, like dense grains (such as brown rice) that can carry you through the day by satisfying your body's needs.

• Exercise! It's the key to permanent weight control. Exercising before a meal will *increase* your metabolism and *decrease* your appetite, often for several hours afterwards.

#3 Sugar craving and blood sugar imbalances.

Some dieters drastically lower their fats, but then replace them with empty carbohydrates, like sugars and starches. Sugar binging is a common result of the overeating/non-eating diet pattern. Sugar provides a temporary "insulin rush," but is then followed by a powerful craving for more food as blood sugar drops. Sugar bingers routinely eat 60 to 70% more calories the following meal. Few calories are burned after a sugar binge because raised insulin levels mean more calories are transformed into fat.

"Grazing" (eating several small highly nutritious meals throughout the day) often works for sugar cravers. Sugar dieters who only eat one meal may steadily *gain weight*, because the foods in that one meal often contain three or four times more calories and fat than fresh "grazing" foods.

Signs of sugar craving and blood sugar imbalances:
• mood swings, frequent anger or crying spells.
• fatigue after eating, especially after dessert or sweet foods.
• having a wired feeling that is only relieved by eating sweets.

A low glycemic diet is another good answer for sugar cravers. A low-glycemic diet keeps insulin levels low so fewer calories are turned into fat and more are burned for energy. By combining low glycemic foods, like high fiber foods, and exercise with certain nutritional supplements, you can also optimize brain biochemistry, so that as a dieter you'll feel more comfortable while dieting, and can diet without binging.

What is a low glycemic diet? Whole, natural foods usually have a low-glycemic index. They don't elevate blood sugar after a meal. High-glycemic index foods, like sugary foods, put blood sugar on a roller coaster, elevating it too rapidly. Insulin responds immediately to stimulate fat production and storage. Too much insulin also causes too much sugar storage, resulting in low blood sugar. Low blood sugar causes stress hormone release, fatigue and ultimately ravenous hunger.

Plant fiber regulates digestion for more balanced blood sugar levels. Plant fiber binds with most fats to prevent their absorption. In addition, plant fiber foods speed up bowel transit time to take stress off your liver so it can metabolize fats efficiently.

When you add more plant fiber to your diet, you'll have less cravings for sugar.

Note: Some spices decrease sugar cravings. Spices like cinnamon, clove and bay leaf help control both blood sugar levels and sugar cravings.

Herbal supplements for sugar cravers fall into three categories -
1) herbs to reduce sugar cravings;
2) herbs to balance low blood sugar (hypoglycemia);
3) herbs to balance high blood sugar (latent diabetes).

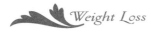

Herbal balancing supplements for sugar cravers:

•Ginseng is a key herb for regulating blood sugar to control sugar cravings. I combine it with licorice in a GINSENG/LICORICE ELIXIR™ for maximum sugar stabilizing.

•A fiber-rich herbal drink, like Crystal Star's LIGHT WEIGHT™ Herbal Diet Plan™, can reduce sugar cravings and build a protein "floor" under a blood sugar drop.

-Note: If you are hypoglycemic, add a sugar stabilizing compound for low blood sugar like Crystal Star's SUGAR STRATEGY LOW™.

-Note: If you have a tendency to latent diabetes, add a sugar stabilizing compound for high blood sugar like Crystal Star's SUGAR STRATEGY HIGH™.

Other sugar balancing supplements to consider:

• *Spirulina* - a craving for sweets may indicate that your body really needs more protein. Green protein from spirulina can relieve sweet cravings with a daily supplement.

• Other "supergreen foods" also help. An afternoon green drink can help ease a craving for sweets. I have used PROGREENS by NutriCology, GREEN MAGMA by Green Foods, and VITALITY SUPERGREEN by Body Ecology with success.

• *Bee pollen and royal jelly* also provide protein energy, amino acids and pantothenic acid for adrenal stimulation. (Or take 2000mg *pantothenic acid*, with *chromium picolinate* 200mcg daily.)

• *Gymnema sylvestre* caps before meals modulate sugar assimilation in the bloodstream.

• *Alpha-lipoic acid* improves body response to insulin and increases its use of carbohydrates as fuel. For appetite control, take two 300mg tabs before breakfast, and another tab before dinner. Continue for 1 month until your appetite for sweets lessens. Then take 1 tab at breakfast and one at dinner for 1 month.

Diet tips for sugar cravings and blood sugar imbalance:
- Make a conscious decision to resist eating sugary foods. (As a former "chocoholic," I know how hard this temptation is.... but the rewards of a balanced body are worth it.)

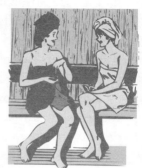

- Hyperthermia helps. Dieters taking a dry sauna 2 to 3 times a week have more balanced blood sugar levels and less sugar cravings than dieters that don't.

- Try *stevia rebaudiana*, a sweet leafy herb used as a natural sweetener in South America for over 1500 years. Known as "sweet herb," *stevia* has been highly controversial since the FDA virtually banned its use in this country (after heavy lobbying by the Nutra-Sweet industry) in 1991. Suspicion that the ban was heavily influenced by Nutra-Sweet interests finally became so public, and the instances of serious illness involved with Nutra-Sweet so common, (*more than any other food additive in U.S. history*), that stevia has now been returned to American markets. Clinical studies indicate that *stevia* is safe to use even in cases of severe sugar imbalance.

Research shows that *stevia* can actually regulate blood sugar. In South America, *stevia* is sold as therapy to people with diabetes and hypoglycemia. Studies also show that *stevia* lowers high blood pressure but does not affect normal blood pressure.

A refined Japanese product, called Stevioside, made from *stevia* leaf, is 300 times sweeter than sugar, and is currently used everywhere (except the U.S.) as a natural sweetener. However, while Stevioside does not affect blood glucose levels and works safely for both diabetics and hypoglycemics, it does not retain the extraordinary healing benefits of whole *stevia* leaf.

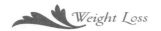

Stevia is effective for weight control because it contains no calories, yet significantly increases glucose tolerance and inhibits glucose absorption. **Sugar cravers benefit the most from stevia,** reporting that it decreases their desire for sugary foods, as well as their desire for tobacco and alcoholic beverages. For sugar-cravers' weight loss, use *stevia* as a sugar substitute when you can.

Stevia is approximately 25 times sweeter than sugar when made as an infusion with 1 tsp. leaves to 1 cup of water. *Two drops of the infusion equal 1 teaspoon of sugar in sweetness.* In baking, 1 teasp. of stevia powder equals 1 cup of sugar.

Note: A facial mask of water-based *stevia* extract effectively smooths out skin wrinkles and heals skin blemishes, including acne. Apply a drop of the extract directly on a blemish outbreak. Experts say that *stevia* may soon be regarded as one of the most "good for you" sweeteners on earth.

#4 Liver malfunction and cellulite formation.

Liver malfunction is directly connected to sugar metabolism as a cause of weight problems. When the liver is working poorly, the blood becomes sugar-saturated, overly stressing the pancreas, inviting diabetes. Hypoglycemic attacks are due not only to improper insulin response, but also to a sluggish liver.

Cellulite, a result of poorly metabolized fats, especially saturated fats, is a weight problem compounded by weak liver function. (See cellulite section in this booklet for specifics.)

A healthy liver is vital for successful weight loss, because the liver is responsible for fat metabolism, as well as for carbohydrates and protein metabolism.

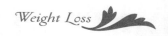

Signs of liver malfunction:
- great tiredness
- unexplained weight gain
- poor digestion
- unexplained depression or melancholy
- PMS
- food and chemical sensitivities
- chronic constipation/indigestion unrelieved by antacids
- a man who is thin everywhere else, but who has a protruding stomach often has an enlarged liver

Herbs can be primary therapy for a sluggish liver.

• "Bitters" herbs like Crystal Star's BITTERS & LEMON™ extract or SWEETISH BITTERS ELIXIR by Gaia Herbs, are a key to liver cleansing. They revitalize digestive functions by enhancing secretions of the liver, pancreas, stomach, and small intestine, improve nutrient absorption and protect the liver from endogenous toxins.

• MILK THISTLE SEED extract may be used for long term liver support, because it's gentle, and optimizes other liver cleansing choices.

Other liver supplements that help fat metabolism include:
• Crystal Star amino/enzyme formula AMINO ZYME™.
• Bee pollen and royal jelly for amino acids and B vitamins.
• Lipotropics like lecithin, choline, inositol and methionine to break down and liquefy fats on the digestive level.
• Vitamin B complex to assist with liver detoxification and fat metabolism. I especially like Nature's Secret ULTIMATE B.
• *DANDELION BURDOCK* formula by Rosemary Gladstar (available from Frontier Natural Products).

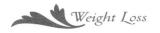

Diet tips for liver malfunction and cellulite formation.

Fried fats and refined sugars compromise your liver health more than any other foods. If you have gone overboard on this type of food, I recommend a quick fat-and-sugar detox to put you back on track for successful weight management.

A quick 24 hour detox to remove excess fats and sugars:

Start the night before with a green leafy salad to "sweep" your bowels. Dry brush your skin before you go to bed to open your pores for the night's cleansing eliminations. Then detox the next 24 hours with fresh juices, pure water, and a long walk during the day.

Upon rising: have a cup of green tea to cut through and eliminate fatty wastes.

Mid-morning: have a cup of apple juice to rebalance and restore normal pH.

Lunch: enjoy a mixed vegetable juice - a must for your detox program. (Make it from scratch or find one you like at your health food store or juice bar. Even regular V-8 juice works just fine.) Vegetables are nature's sweepers and scourers, cleaning out your body like no other food can.

Mid-afternoon: take a glass of papaya/pineapple juice to enhance enzyme production.

Dinner: have some miso soup to alkalize body chemistry and enhance immunity.

After dinner: relax with a cup of your favorite herbal tea. The liver works overtime at night to digest fats. A "constitutional" walk in the evening after dinner or just before retiring really helps stimulate liver activity.

Note: After your detox, concentrate on keeping fats and sugars low in your diet to reduce cravings for them.

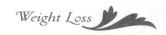

#5 Poor circulation and low energy

For some dieters, initial weight loss is rapid, but then a plateau is reached and further weight loss becomes difficult because restricted food intake slows down metabolism. Herbal combinations help reactivate metabolism, convert stored fat to energy, and boost circulation to help a dieter get over plateaus.

Signs of poor circulation: • hands and feet becoming cold easily • poor memory • ringing in the ears.

Boost your circulation and energy with herbal therapy.

Herbs like hawthorn, ginkgo biloba and ginger recharge your energy and circulation; or an herb tea with metabolism-activating herbs like Crystal Star RAINFOREST ENERGY™ tea.

Ginseng formulas are a key for both low energy and circulation. Consider an herbal formula like Crystal Star's GINSENG SIX™. An adrenal activator like Crystal Star's ADRN-ACTIVE™ addresses glandular energy for long term results.

Other energy and circulation supplements include:
• CoQ_{10}, - 60mg daily for anti-oxidant enzyme activity.
• Amino acids *glutamine* and *carnitine*, 500mg each daily.
• LIVING ENERGY tabs by Futurebiotics
• Nature's Path TRACE-LYTE mineral electrolytes. By restoring electrolyte balance, energy circuits are switched back on.
• For circulation stimulation - BUTCHER'S BROOM caps by Rosemary Gladstar, or CIRCUPLEX by Futurebiotics.

Diet tips for poor circulation and low energy:
• Sip on hot broths to speed up circulation. Add garlic, cayenne pepper or horseradish for an extra circulation boost.
• Regular massage helps restore good circulation.

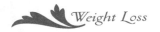

#6 Poor elimination... detoxing bowel and bladder.

Chronic constipation affects more than 30 million Americans! Over 75% of American women are affected by bladder and kidney elimination problems at least once a decade!

In times past, rich foods like red meats, rich cheeses, cream, butter, sugars and sweets were reserved for festive occasions. Today, people make them a part of every meal. Although the fat and sugar make them delicious, the reality is that these foods are low in nutrition and very hard to eliminate. Environmental agents like pollutants, pesticides, and chemicals that appear in these foods obstruct body processes.

Nowhere are these lifestyle facts more evident or more frustrating than in our national weight control problem.

Enzymes are a key to elimination for weight control.

Enzymes handle digestion and speed up digestion of foods that the body tends to store, like fats (the enzyme lipase works specifically to digest fats). Enzymes keep your entire digestive tract free of waste build-up.

Enzymes in fresh vegetables are the best foods to eat for a free flowing body and healthy elimination. Unfortunately, Americans eat less fruits and vegetables than any other society. **America is a staggeringly enzyme-deficient nation.**

Let me share with you a quick method I have used with hundreds of people to determine enzyme activity and supply. It's a cheese test.

1) Cut up a serving size piece of cheese into a salad. Eat the salad and notice your digestion. Is it easy? Do you feel bloated or gassy? Do you feel too full?

2) The next day, fix yourself a grilled cheese sandwich so that the cheese is heated and melts. Eat the sandwich and notice your digestion. Do you have indigestion? Do you feel bloated or gassy? Do you feel full long after you eat? Are you constipated the next morning?

If you answer yes to these questions, you aren't getting enough enzymes to process or eliminate your food very well.

Signs of bowel and bladder elimination problems:
• frequent bad breath and body odor;
• infrequent bowel movements;
• coated tongue.

Herbal cleansers can help reactivate normal elimination and body functions. An herbal tea formula like Crystal Star's LEAN & CLEAN™ DIET tea provides weight loss cleansing support for elimination problems.

A therapeutic bath like Crystal Star's POUNDS OFF™ bath starts a cleansing sweat in about 15 minutes. Take it once a week to release toxins the easy way.

Other elimination aid supplements include:
•Flax seed oil, 2 teasp. daily for essential fatty acids.
•Acidophilus, for more efficient digestive processes.
•Green superfood tablets, like Nature's Secret ULTIMATE GREEN™ for better kidney and colon function.
•An herbal cleanser like Crystal Star's FIBER & HERBS CLEANSE™ caps.
•Nature's Secret ULTIMATE CLEANSE.
•Ethical Nutrients 20 DAY DETOX DIGESTIVE SYSTEM.
•Transformation Enzyme Corp. BALANCE ZYME PLUS.

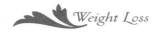

What about exercise? Can it really make your body a fat-burning machine? Before age 19, you can still increase or decrease the number of fat cells in your body. However at 20, that number no longer changes. Losing weight after 20 means shrinking existing fat cell size. You can shrink fat cells by exercising. Here's how it works. 30 minutes of aerobic exercise increases adrenaline production which, in turn, causes fat cells to release fat into the bloodstream. The muscles then pick up the fat to use for a quick source of energy. As your fat cells shrink, you become thinner, more fit and healthy.

Calculate your body fat. Ideal body fat for women is between 16-25%. For men, it's between 10-15%.

Here's how to determine your body fat.

• Measure your height and the widest portion of your hips to the nearest half-inch.

• Using the chart below, run a diagonal line between your hip girth and height.

• The number you intersect at is your percentage of body fat. When a man's body fat exceeds 25% and a woman's exceeds 32%, he or she is considered clinically obese.

HIPS (inches)	% BODY FAT	HEIGHT (inches)
-32-	-10-	-72-
-	-	-
-34-	-14-	-70-
-	-	-
-36-	-18-	-68-
-	-	-
-38-	-22-	-66-
-	-	-
-40-	-26-	-64-
-	-	-
-42-	-30-	-62-
-	-	-
44	-34-	-60-
-	-	-
46	-38-	-58-
-	-	-
48	-42-	-56-

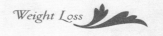

Men & Women Have Different Needs For Weight Control

It's no secret that men and women have different body make-ups.
You can use this fact to better target your weight loss program.

About women and fat:

Women have a gynoid pattern of fat distribution that accumulates fat around the hips and buttocks. It is much harder for women to lose fat in their problem areas than for men.

Estrogen in the female body directs the storage of "sex-specific fat", on the buttocks, hips and thighs for the purposes of child-bearing and hormone functions. As women get older, the problem escalates.

Estrogen reduction during menopause contributes another change in fat distribution. Menopausal women develop more fat storage in the deep abdominal cavity than menstruating women. The good news is that small changes in diet and lifestyle can help solve the weight problems that women have.

I recommend that women approach weight control on two fronts for the best results. 1) Increase your metabolism to burn more fat (especially after menopause). 2) Make aerobic exercise part of your regular diet program.

You can recharge your metabolism through your diet. Sea vegetables work for women to recharge metabolism and balance thyroid activity against many menopausal hormone problems and body changes (including body thickening) .

I like toasted nori, wakame, kombu and sweet sea palm with their natural iodine, potassium, B vitamins and bioflavonoids. Two chopped, dried tablespoons are a natural therapeutic dose.

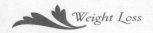
Just add them to any salad, soup or pizza. Sea veggies are available at Oriental markets and health food stores. I also recommend eating at least 6 pieces of sushi (any kind) twice a week.

Thermogenic herbs can boost fat burning activity. Thermogenesis is the process by which the body produces heat from stored calories in brown adipose tissue (BAT). Increasing thermogenesis means getting rid of calories not used by the body.

Some women with low thermogenesis store too many unused calories as fat instead of burning them off. Thermogenic herbs can help these women get over the hump during a weight control program. We also know that stimulating thermogenesis can actually help reduce fat tissue. In contrast, a very low-calorie diet may cause the body to lose fat-burning, lean muscle tissue when it interprets fewer calories as a signal for famine and turns to muscle for fuel.

I recommend Crystal Star Herbal Nutrition's THERMO-CITRIN® GINSENG™ caps with garcinia cambogia and other thermogenic herbs like spirulina, sida cordifolia, panax ginseng, green tea, guarana and capsicum. I have also worked with ELIM/SLIM SUPREME by Gaia Herbs, with good results.

Here are some more tried and true watchwords:
• The amino acid ornithine (500mg daily) helps women boost metabolism and curb appetite.

• Eat only when you're hungry. Women who eat when they're stressed or depressed tend to overeat.

• Eat more whole foods, in their natural, unprocessed state. Especially eat nutritious foods, like brown rice at lunchtime. It

will help carry a woman's body through the day by providing B vitamins and minerals for low fat, foundation energy.

• Deep breathing for women. It may sound too easy, but it's true. Breathing processes 70% of the body's wastes. Shallow breathing slows down metabolism as well as detoxification. Breathing deep from the abdomen will deliver oxygen to your cells, help get rid of fat, increase your energy and boost metabolism. It also helps regulate heart rate, lower blood pressure and improve immune response.

• Try aromatherapy. New research shows that the smell of banana, green apple and peppermint can help reduce weight!

• Get aerobic! Aerobic exercise combined with a low fat, low cal, fresh foods diet is particularly good for women. No long term weight control plan will work without it and with it, almost every plan will. One study found that overweight women who cut their calories and added an aerobic exercise program had significantly less PMS problems such as mood swings and poor concentration. They also had lower blood levels of monoamine oxidase, an enzyme linked to PMS, and they lost an average of 36 pounds.

I like taking brisk walks after dinner because it helps boost nighttime liver activity for fat metabolism. (The liver metabolizes fats and dumps a lot of its wastes at night.). It may also help you live longer. A new study in the *Journal of the American Medical Association* revealed that taking just 6 brisk, half-hour walks *a month* cuts risk of death 44%, compared to people who do not exercise.

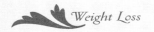
About men and fat:

Men have android fat patterns that tend to be distributed in the abdomen area. In other words, guys get potbellies! There are two types of fat, subcutaneous and visceral. A man with a hard potbelly has more visceral fat (fat that lies between the muscles and organs). Soft bellies are largely comprised of subcutaneous fat which lies just beneath the skin and is harder to get rid of. Men have more visceral fat than women; it's one of the reasons why they seem to be able to shake extra pounds easier than women. The bad news is that hard bellies formed from visceral fat are linked to cardiovascular diseases and intestinal problems. Reducing fatty foods and exercising regularly is a solution that usually works for men.

Here are some tips to help men manage weight problems.

• Control your portions so you don't overeat. It's a big problem for American men who are encouraged to dig in to second, even third helpings as a sign of manliness, or approval for the cook. Overeating happens when you eat lots of highly processed, chemical-laced foods, and junk food snacks that don't have much nutrition to help you feel full.

Men also tend to overeat when they're under stress or on-the-run.... circumstances under which many American men eat.

• Drink plenty of water to naturally suppress appetite and maintain a good metabolic rate.

• Enzymes really work for men as a weight loss technique. I have worked with men who were not able to assimilate their food well, or who ate lots of processed foods their bodies didn't use, and became overeaters.

Take enzymes with meals to help prevent gas, heartburn and indigestion naturally. In my experience, enzymes work far better than antacids. They speed up digestion and keep the entire digestive tract free of waste build-up. The best enzymes come from fresh plant foods. Cooking largely destroys them. So have a fresh salad at least once a day for weight control. And if you can't make them, take them. I regularly recommend Nature's Secret REZYME to men with success.

• Eat more whole foods in their natural, unprocessed state. I regularly recommend to men that they eat extra fruits in the morning because they offer a blood sugar-raising glycogen energy punch, are easily digested and ensure regularity.

• Exercise is one of the main pillars of weight control for men.... even more than women. Exercising just 25 to 30 minutes a day will help you lose about 20 pounds a year, improve your energy and stamina, recharge your cardiovascular health and increase your life span!

• Metabolism, the process by which you burn calories, slows down once you get past forty, but you can reactivate it. In men, calorie-burning metabolism is most affected by lean muscle mass. **The more muscle you have, the better your metabolism rate.** In one study, men who participated in intense strength training exercise had an elevated metabolism for 15 hours after their workout!

Incorporate some weight bearing exercise into your exercise program, but be reasonable about it. Many weight bearing exercise injuries are the result of over-zealousness.... trying to lift too much weight, lifting the wrong way or simply lifting for too long. Start slow and stick with it.

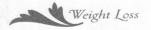
•Spices like cinnamon, cayenne, mustard and ginger can speed up a man's fat burning process. The amino acid arginine (1000mg daily) is also a useful tool for men trying to reactivate metabolism, because it supports more lean muscle mass.

•Poor liver health contributes to a pot belly. Your liver is your primary fat metabolizing organ. Did you know that a man who is thin everywhere else but has a protruding stomach often has an enlarged liver?

You can help restore your liver with natural remedies. Here are some tips:

Drink green tea, about 2 cups a day in the morning and early afternoon, to optimize your liver's ability to digest excess fats. Green tea changes the metabolic pattern of the liver by changing the ratio of two metabolic enzymes, cytochrome P450 and glucuronyltransferase, to help the body excrete toxins and fatty wastes. Moreover, green tea has been found to protect against cancers of the lungs, skin, liver, pancreas, and stomach, protect the heart, lower cholesterol and regulate blood sugar and insulin levels. Green tea is also a gentle cleanser which leaves you feeling refreshed and invigorated.

I also recommend *milk thistle seed* extract for long term liver support. Ten to 15 drops for a period of 1 to 3 months, gently cleanses the liver and improves its function. More than 300 studies show that *silymarin*, one of *milk thistle's* constituents, can prevent toxins from even entering the liver and can actually increase the liver's ability to generate new, healthy cells.

Take your B vitamins. Deficiencies in B-complex can cause problems with the metabolism of fats and carbohydrates.

Weight Control After 40

There's no doubt about it. Weight loss gets more difficult after 40. **The latest figures show that a person's body fat typically doubles between the ages of 20 and 50.** Everybody goes

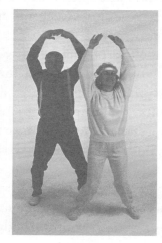

through a change
mone changes of
affect our body
both men and
the worst prob-
ness oriented
as they reach
50's is a discon-
ening and a slow,
weight. It seems
erybody, even for
always been slim,
diet, and who

of life. The hor-
our middle years
shapes, too......for
women. One of
lems America's fit-
population faces
their late 40's and
certing body thick-
steady rise in
to happen with ev-
people who have
who have a good
regularly exercise.

What's going on here?

For women, a primary calorie-burning process grinds to a halt after menopause. A woman's menstrual cycle consumes extra calories. Some experts theorize that the metabolic rise in the last two weeks of the menstrual cycle accounts for 15,000-20,000 calories per year. Those calories can really start to add up when menstruation ceases, so these women tend to have more fat and less lean muscle tissue than women who are still menstruating.

While a woman may need to work a little harder to lose that extra fat later in life, once her body adjusts to its new hormone levels, weight gain stabilizes, becomes more manageable, and in many cases, falls back to pre-menopause levels.

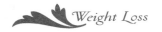

Changes in estrogen levels for women and testosterone levels for men mean that our body chemistry is in transition. Clearly, metabolic rates slow as we age, so it takes food longer to digest, and more of it goes into storage. Our bodies begin to lose the ability to break down and use large quantities of fat. People who could always lose weight when they were younger just by going on a crash diet for a weekend or a week find that strategy doesn't work anymore.

Most of us become less physically active as we age, which leads to muscle loss, an important factor for a youthful body. Still, achieving your proper weight is a goal worth pursuing. The newest studies show that gaining even just a few pounds as we age lowers life expectancy and raises heart attack risk by up to 50%! Increases in body fat are also linked to colon, prostate and breast cancers.

Can we solve age-related weight problems? Can we modify our diets and lifestyles to retain a youthful body as we age? Weight control solutions have to be approached differently when metabolism slows down. Just eating all the low fat or even fat free foods available today doesn't seem to make a difference. Artificial sweeteners don't keep sugar dieting on track, either. In fact, the newest studies show that a significant number of people compensate for not eating sweets by eating more fat to improve the taste of their foods.

Do we all go through a change of life? Nature seems to have a variety of health reasons for body shape changes, from cancer protection to bone preservation. Logically knowing the reasons, of course, doesn't satisfy the youthful equation. The good news is that we can do something about our weight, our body tone and our looks.

I have been working for several years to develop natural weight control techniques for people trying to maintain healthy body weight and tone after their metabolism changes. The program shows promise and results.

For weight loss after 40, begin with two starting points:
1) Improve body chemistry at the gland and hormone level.
2) Re-establish better, long-lasting metabolic rates.

Natural, effective techniques to boost metabolism after 40:

#1 LOVE YOUR LIVER.
The liver is your body's chemical plant responsible for fat metabolism. It is also intricately involved with the hormone functions of the body, so it is the prime target to optimize for weight loss after 40. Weight gain and energy loss are often the result of a liver which has become enlarged through overwork, alcohol exhaustion and congestion.

• Ginseng compounds help improve body chemistry.
• Ginseng supports every area of fat and sugar metabolism, especially those involved with the liver.
• Ginseng contains phyto-hormones to balance estrogen levels in women and to normalize testosterone levels in men.
• Ginseng improves digestion for better nutrient use, and less food storage.
• Ginseng energizes the body so you don't eat as much.
• Ginseng enhances thermogenesis by helping re-activate metabolism, and extending the effects of other thermogenic herbs.
A good thermogenesis (calorie-burning) herbal formula with ginseng works extremely well. I have used Crystal Star's THERMO-GINSENG™ extract for many years with success.

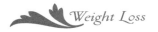

#2 CONSCIOUSLY EAT LESS.

As metabolism slows, you don't need to fuel it up as much, because your body doesn't use up the nutrients like it once did. If you eat like you did in your 20's and 30's, your body will store too much, mostly as fat.

- **Make sure you are eating a low fat diet.**

Even with all the fat-conscious foods on the market today, Americans still consume one-third of their calories as fat. Your fat intake should be about 20% for weight control, 15% or less for weight loss.

But remember: no-fat is not good for weight loss, either.

Your body goes into a survival mode if you eliminate all fat, shedding it's highly active lean muscle tissue to reduce the body's need for food. When lean muscle tissue decreases, fat burning slows or stops.

- **Control your food portions.**

Portion control is a cornerstone of weight control. Even though your diet is healthy and the foods you eat reasonably low in fat, there's no way you can eat all you want of anything.

A recent study by researchers at Tufts University compared the metabolism of 16 women, half in their 20's and the rest older than 60. They discovered that older women burned only 70% as much fat after eating large meals as the younger women.

I recommend eating smaller meals every two to three hours to keep your appetite hole from gnawing, and to keep metabolic rate high. Small meals virtually prevent carbohydrates and proteins from being converted into fat.

New research shows that moderate food intake may extend lifespan by as much as ten years!

• **Control hunger with safe herbal appetite suppressants.**
Herbs offer good choices for keeping our bodies in the manner to which we are accustomed. Herbal weight loss combinations help because they can address almost every individual problem of weight control. And they're slow and steady, with a long history of effectiveness.

Superfood herbs like barley grass, spirulina, sea vegetables and alfalfa can be a key to controlling appetite. A green drink made with these extremely low-calorie foods may be used between meals to rapidly decrease the craving for high-calorie foods. Compounds with herbs like Crystal Star's ENERGY GREEN™ drink can raise both metabolic rate and activity levels.

#3 RAISE YOUR METABOLISM.
A higher metabolic rate means you burn more fat, lose weight easier, and maintain your ideal body weight more comfortably.

• **Don't skip meals.....especially breakfast.**
People skip breakfast because it's so easy to rush out the door to work and not miss it. But breakfast is the worst meal to skip if you want to raise metabolism. It sends a temporary fasting signal to the brain that food is going to be scarce. So stress hormones increase, and the body begins shedding lean muscle tissue in order to decrease its need for food.

By the time you eat again, your pancreas is so sensitized to a lack of food, that it sharply increases blood insulin levels, the body's signal to make fat.

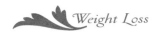

- **Reduce both sugars and fats - they slow metabolism.**

Fats have twice the calories, gram for gram, as protein and complex carbohydrates. They also use only 2% of their calories before the fat storage process begins. Protein and carbohydrates burn almost 25% of their calories before storing them as fat.

Limit alcohol consumption, even wine, to two glasses or less a day. With seven calories per gram, alcohol sugars shift metabolism in favor of fat depositing; too much alcohol burdens the liver and stimulates the appetite.

- **Eat fat-burning foods.**

Foods that raise metabolism are fresh fruits and vegetables (full of enzymes), whole grains and legumes. Eat fruits for breakfast or between meals. If you eat them with or after meals, the fructose is likely to be converted to fat by the liver. Eat early in the day to lose weight, when your metabolism is at its best, and when you have hours of activity ahead of you to burn fats.

Note: Sea vegetables work especially well for women to recharge metabolism and balance thyroid activity against many hormone problems after menopause begins. I like toasted nori, wakame, kombu and sweet sea palm, to recharge metabolism with natural iodine and potassium after menopause. Two tablespoons are a therapeutic dose. Add them chopped and dried to any salad, soup, rice dish or omelet. If you like sushi, add 6 or more pieces (any kind), twice a week to your diet.

- **Re-activate your fat-burning systems with herbs.**

Use herbs to stoke your metabolic fire. A broad spectrum formula with herbal adaptogens like *panax and Siberian ginsengs, suma, gotu kola, and licorice root,* help balance the body's homeostasis; *ginkgo biloba and hawthorn* boost circulation; *bee pollen, alfalfa,* and phytohormone-containing herbs like *sarsaparilla and black cohosh* support the liver; spices and sea vegetables like *cayenne, ginger, kelp and spirulina* help the thyroid gland, which governs metabolism. I recommend FEEL GREAT™ caps by Crystal Star Herbal Nutrition as a whole body tonic to enhance fat burning and well-being.

- **Amino acids to boost metabolism and keep lean muscle.**
  —L-Phenylalanine (LPA), suppresses appetite, boosts energy and reduces food craving. (Avoid phenylalanine if you are taking anti-depressant medication, have high blood pressure, are pregnant or have phenylketonuria.)
  —L-Tyrosine is a thyroid precursor and reduces appetite.
  —L-Carnitine suppresses appetite, accelerates fat metabolism and helps control sugar levels.

  Amino acids and appetite-control herbs combined in a formula like Crystal Star's AMINO ZYME™ work extremely well. Other amino acid metabolic products I have worked with to assist weight maintenance include MYOPLEX LITE by EAS, and AMINO BALANCE by Anabol Naturals.

- **Drink plenty of water.**
  Water naturally suppresses appetite, helps maintain a high metabolic rate, and **actually reduces fat deposits.** In fact, water may be the most important catalyst for increased fat burning, because it increases the liver's main functions of detoxification and metabolism to process more fats. Don't be concerned with fluid retention. High water intake actually decreases bloating, because it flushes out sodium and toxins. **Studies show that decreasing water intake causes increased fat deposits.** Expert dieters drink eight glasses of water a day. They know each pound of fat burned releases 22 ounces of water which must be flushed away along with the metabolic by-products of fat breakdown.

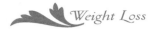
• **Get moderate doses of sunlight.**

The sun receives a lot of criticism today, but sunlight in moderation increases metabolism and food digestion. One of the best choices is to eat outdoors. Sunlight can produce metabolic effects in the body similar to that of physical training.

#4 EXERCISE FOR SURE.

Daily exercise is the key to permanent, painless weight control. No diet will work without exercise; with it, almost every diet will.

Exercise before a meal raises blood sugar levels, increases metabolism and decreases appetite, often for hours afterward.

Even if you just slightly change your eating habits, you can still lose weight with a brisk hour's walk, or 15 minutes of aerobic exercise.

Aerobic exercise, combined with a low fat, low calorie, fresh foods diet is particularly good for women. One study found that overweight women who cut their calories and added an aerobic exercise program significantly reduced their PMS problems like mood swings and poor concentration. They also had lower blood levels of monoamine oxidase (an enzyme linked to PMS)..... and they lost an average of 36 pounds.

Here's how cutting down even moderately on fatty, sugary foods, and adding exercise provides the body look we all want:

• One pound of fat represents 3500 calories. A 3 mile walk burns 250 calories. After 2 weeks of walking you will have lost a pound of real fat. That amounts to 3 pounds a month or 30 pounds a year - all without starving.

• Exercise also promotes an "afterburn" effect, raising the

metabolic rate from 1.00 up to between 1.05 and 1.15 per minute for up to 24 hours afterwards. Your calories are used up at an even faster rate *after* you exercise.

The biggest exercise problem is the dropout level. People quit altogether if they overdo it. But you don't have to overdo it to lose weight.

In fact, walking is considered to be superior to running as a fat-burning exercise, and it keeps your metabolic rate high for hours afterwards. An exercise heart rate around 60% of the maximum burns mostly fat. *Intense exercise* that causes the heart rate to rise over 80% of the maximum actually decreases metabolism, because it burns muscle tissue instead of fat.

Studies on walking and weight loss show that, in test groups who walked at different rates for six months or more, **the slowest walking group lost the most weight.** Kinda blows a hole in the old excuse that exercise is too hard, right?

Exercise builds and maintains your lean muscle. Loss of calorie-gobbling lean muscle tissue almost guarantees that you'll gain back any weight you've lost. **Pound for pound, lean muscle burns five times as many calories as other body tissue.**

Adding just 10 pounds of lean muscle can burn 600 calories per day. You would have to run six miles a day, seven days a week to burn the same number of calories. In fact, 10 pounds of lean muscle tissue can burn one pound of fat per week, 52 pounds of fat per year. The best way to increase lean muscle mass is through resistance training, or weight lifting.

However, I recommend that you choose an activity that you enjoy and will stick to. Swimming, biking and hiking are all good alternatives to weight training.

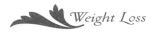

It is easier for men to lose weight than women, but men, too, face challenges with weight gain as they grow older. Men consume more of their calories from fatty foods (like hamburgers and sausage) than women, so exercise is a necessity for their weight control. Colon cancer, strongly linked to excessive fat intake, is one of the leading causes of death in men. Sometimes it takes a major medical setback later in life from a weight problem for a man to get on a "fit body" program.

I believe exercise is a nutrient in itself. Exercise can give you more energy and stamina, better cardiovascular health, an improved self-image and increased longevity. When you begin an exercise program, you may notice skin eruptions, body odor or bad breath. These are usually signs that the body is clearing out congested wastes and will normally disappear within a short time. Whatever exercise program you choose for weight management and better health, start slow and stick with it.

Thermogenesis is Critical To Weight Loss After 40.

Thermogenesis is about fat burning.
About 75% of the calories you eat work to keep you alive and support your resting metabolic rate. The rest can be stored as white fat, or burned up by special body cells known as brown adipose tissue, or BAT.

Brown fat tissue is really a fat-burning factory, burning up calories your body doesn't need, a process called thermogenesis.

Brown fat is the body's chief regulator of thermogenesis, so the more active your brown fat is, the easier it is to maintain a desirable weight.

Dieters who rely solely on calorie restriction usually end up disappointed with the results, because extreme caloric restriction lowers the rate of thermogenesis. **Your body actually burns less fat than it did before you started dieting.**

People who yo-yo on and off low calorie diets have more problems to contend with. When a yo-yo dieter begins to increase calorie intake after dieting, their metabolic rate does not return to pre-diet levels, so they store more calories as fat than they did before they started!

Too much fat-making means too little thermogenesis. Everybody increases metabolism after eating, a process known as diet-induced thermogenesis. But the amounts of heat vary widely. Lean people experience a 40% increase in heat production after a meal. Overweight people may have only an increase of 10%. Obesity occurs primarily when brown fat isn't working properly, only a little thermogenesis takes place, and the body deals with the excess calories by storing them as fat. This is normally what's happening in the phenomenon known as middle-aged spread. During our mid-life years, starting in our late 30's and early 40's, a genetic timer shuts down the thermogenic mechanism. Turning this timer back on is the secret to re-activating thermogenesis and a more youthful metabolism.

Research into the genetic basis of obesity shows that some people are not born with enough brown fat. People who eat lightly but still can't lose weight, gain even more weight at middle age because the little brown fat they did have is reduced even further. Thermogenesis research, however, demonstrates that it is possible to reverse the genetic fault responsible for obesity

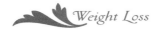

in some of these people. Natural thermogenesis stimulants like certain herbs, have been successful at reactivating brown fat in middle age.

What is brown fat? Brown fat is present in the body in much smaller quantities than white or storage fat. It's located only in certain places - between the shoulder blades, in the armpits, on the back of the neck and surrounding the large blood vessels in the chest and abdomen. It can be stimulated to help the body convert white fat back into calories that can then be disposed of through thermal combustion. This is how, for instance, the herbal spa body wraps work.

Here's how brown fat works to stimulate thermogenesis.
A special protein, called uncoupling protein, breaks down, or uncouples, the train of biochemical events that the cells use to turn calories into energy. Sometimes, even though the uncoupling protein produces heat, the resulting energy may not go anywhere, so thermogenesis doesn't happen.

Brown fat cells, however, continue to convert calories into heat as long as they are stimulated, and as long as there is white fat for them to work on. Brown fat activity is also self-perpetuating, because it energizes more uncoupling proteins, produces more brown fat cells, and results in substantially more excess calories being burned off as heat through thermogenesis.

Note: You may have heard that brown fat can be reactivated by taking cold showers. This information came from early testing which showed that metabolism increased as body temperature dropped. But this technique has proven to be much less effective than either thermogenic stimulating herbal compounds or supplements like HCA.

Thermogenic herbal compounds are one of the best choices for reactivating the process of thermogenesis. Thermogenic herbs can increase calorie burning without additional support of diet changes or exercise, although these things offer additional benefits.

• Thermogenic herbs increase blood flow to lean muscle tissue, so it works faster and longer.

• Thermogenic herbs suppress appetite. You eat less with less effort.

• The longer you take thermogenic herb formulas, the more effective they tend to become, because they help your body produce enough thermogenic activity to make a difference.

Ephedra and thermogenesis? It's effective. Is it really safe?
Ephedra, an herb used safely for centuries as a broncho-dilator for chest congestion, also has thermogenic properties. Many herbal thermogenic products are formulated with ephedra, because tests show that one of its constituents, ephedrine, stimulates metabolic energy and boosts calorie-burning. The advantage of ephedra-based products over calorie-restricted crash dieting is that the body actually loses fat tissue.

Ephedrine acts as an analog to adrenaline, helping to turn on brown fat tissue that has become dormant. But ephedrine is tricky to use because the body sets up natural barriers to prevent what it perceives as wasted energy, and requires high dosages of ephedra to overcome them. **Some ephedra extracts are up to 700% more concentrated than the whole powdered herb.**

Unfortunately, high doses of ephedrine, especially if used in an isolated concentrate, act as a central nervous system stimu-

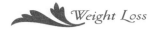

lant, similar to coffee, which sometimes precipitates side effects like increased blood pressure, heart rate, insomnia and anxiety.

Some ephedra products claim to produce euphoria, even ecstasy. These so-called herbally based drugs are generally marketed as "natural" substitutes for illicit street drugs. Of course they have a high potential for safety risks. In fact, most experts acknowledge that ephedra-based products should not be used continuously over a long time because of potential long-term strain on the adrenal glands.

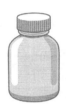 In order to use less ephedrine, some thermogenic weight loss products now combine ephedrine with caffeine and aspirin, about 75mg of ephedrine, 150mg of caffeine, and 300mg of aspirin, claiming that this ratio is effective for weight loss with much less ephedrine. To me, this is a highly stimulative compound with even more dangerous side effects than the original ephedrine. It's the kind of chemical mix that's easy to abuse and over-dose on.

Yet, in my experience, we don't need to make a drug out of ephedra to get the same thermogenic benefits. Whole herb ephedra works just as well as ephedrine, without having to be isolated, concentrated or boosted. Whole herbs are far gentler because they are foods with protective benefits built in. They are far safer and cause less stress on the body.

Whole herb *ephedra*, as it appears in many herbal combinations in health food stores, has proven to stimulate brown fat to burn more white fat. New animal studies show a marked increase in the metabolic rate of brown fat tissue using the whole herb, and it appears that the same will be true for people — addressing the cause of obesity rather than just the symptoms.

In addition, whole herb ephedra has a unique, self-limiting property. As the body adapts to the increased stimulation from ephedra by growing more active brown fat, so its thermogenic need for ephedra's help naturally decreases over time.

I only recommend using whole ephedra, in combination with other whole herbs in expert herbal formulations.

Note: In some states, the Food & Drug Administration has forbidden ephedra to be sold without warnings. Do not use ephedra if you are pregnant, nursing, taking MAO inhibitors or prescription medicines, if you have heart or thyroid disease, prostate enlargement, or diabetes. Ephedra should not to be used by children under 13, unless as a weak tea for broncho-dilation. If you have any pre-existing medical condition, ask your health professional before using ephedra.

Are there other herbal choices that work as well as ephedra without the health unknowns? The answer is yes. There 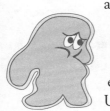 are other brown fat stimulating herbs that don't have heart-speeding effects. *Sida cordifolia*, an Ayurvedic herb, contains a constituent similar to ephedrine that also raises metabolic rate and increases energy, but is far gentler in its action than ephedrine. Undesirable nervousness, insomnia and heart palpitations rarely, if ever, occur with sida cordifolia. Sida cordifolia is especially effective in activating brown fat that has gone dormant from genetic signals due to the process of aging. It's a good answer for weight loss after 40.

I have done a great deal of work with sida cordifolia, and recommend it in thermogenic herbal compounds like Crystal Star's THERMO-CITRIN® GINSENG™ caps.

Other thermogenic, ephedra-free products that I like include PHENSOLUTION by Nature's Secret, and Crystal Star APPE-

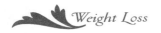

TITE™ caps. Both formulas contain *St. John's Wort*, for positive mood effects while dieting. (Researchers have found that weight loss is directly related to our sense of well being.) The compounds also contain *hawthorn berry* to support the heart and cardiovascular circulation so that you'll lose weight safely.

More choices:

HCA is an herbally-based, natural appetite-suppressant. Hydroxy-Citric Acid, known commercially as CITRIN™ or CITRI-MAX™, comes from the herbal fruit garcinia cambogia. It is an effective aid for holding down appetite in order to lose weight, especially when used with biologically active chromium. Twenty-five years of study indicate that HCA is both safe and effective, especially after metabolism slows down in middle age years. Because of the way in which it works, HCA is also a good choice for overeaters and sugar cravers.

HCA influences three important weight control processes:
- it inhibits the body's fat production and storage;
- it blocks the body's conversion of sugar into fat;
- it controls appetite;
- it increases calorie burning.

The appetite-suppressing action of HCA is different than over-the-counter appetite suppressants, such as phenyl-propanolamine, or prescriptions like amphetamines, meth-amphetamines, fenfluramine, phenmetrazine and di-ethyl-propion. Drugs like these act on the central nervous system, and may lead to depression, nervousness, insomnia, hypertension and rapid heart rate, especially with long term use.

HCA's appetite-suppressing activity works peripherally. It doesn't enter the central nervous system directly, but instead

stimulates an increase in the amount of glycogen that the liver produces to curb appetite. HCA is thus able to inhibit lipogenesis, the process by which the body produces and stores fat. A New York study found that HCA inhibited lipogenesis quickly, within 150 minutes of administration.

Another promising study, conducted by Anthony Conte, M.D., found that HCA from garcinia cambogia, combined with niacin-bound chromium produced an average 11 pound weight reduction in the people studied over an eight-week period.

Can HCA boost thermogenesis, too? The most valuable research on HCA shows that it efficiently activates thermogenesis, preserving lean muscle tissue during fat loss on a reduced-calorie diet. While reducing calories below what it takes to maintain your current weight always causes some lean muscle loss (along with the fat), preserving as much of lean muscle tissue as possible is vital to long-lasting weight control.

Lean muscle can burn calories even at rest while fat tissue is dead weight. Loss of calorie-gobbling lean muscle contributes to the yo-yo syndrome, because your body regains fat tissue on less calories after your diet is over. As with every type of extremely low-calorie diet (below 1200 calories for women and 1500 for men), dieters run the risk of losing too much lean muscle tissue. HCA, along with exercise, helps maintain and build this type of muscle, making it possible to control your weight even with more calories.

A product I have reviewed for effectiveness that contains HCA is ULTIMATE WEIGHT LOSS by Nature's Secret (A two part program containing CRAVELESS and BURNMORE).

• Taking an HCA formula with 500mg of carnitine, and 200mcg of chromium picolinate offers even better results.

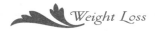

What About Cellulite?

Is liposuction the only answer? Are there natural methods for overcoming this unsightly scourge?

The vast majority of Americans have cellulite. Many people don't need to lose weight as much as they need to lose cellulite. Eighty-six percent of U.S. women over the age of 20 have cellulite deposits on the hips and thighs.

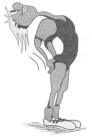 Cellulite affects women far more than men because a woman's skin fibers are thinner and more delicate than a man's. Fatty wastes can become lodged beneath the skin's surface easily in a woman, especially when the liver or lymphatic system is sluggish. Even very thin women have cellulite.

Men are not entirely immune to cellulite. Overweight men get cellulite around the torso and stomach. More than 50% of U.S. men over forty have cellulite deposits on their torso "love handles."

Cellulite is tough to get rid of. Even a good diet and regular exercise may not remove it. Cellulite is composed of waste materials, toxins, water and unmetabolized fats. When the body's circulation and elimination become impaired, connective tissue loses its strength, and unmetabolized fats and wastes become trapped just beneath the skin instead of being expelled through body elimination.

Over a period of time the wastes enlarge, harden and push through spaces in the connective fiber bands that anchor down skin. They cause bulges which appear as dimples, and form the puckering, distorted skin effect we know as cellulite. Skin undulations become apparent as cellulite layers build up.

Unfortunately, this kind of fatty build up is not attached, so it is extremely difficult for the body to process through its elimination channels.

Cellulite tends to form in areas of sluggish circulation, building up where normal cell exchange slows down. While fat is a generalized condition, cellulite deposits settle mainly on the hips, buttocks, thighs and knees. When regular fat is squeezed the skin appears smooth, but cellulite skin ripples like an orange peel, or has the texture of cottage cheese.

Lifestyle factors typically contribute to cellulite formation:
—Excessive dietary chemicals that the body can't process.
—Lack of exercise and a sedentary life-style.
—Hereditary body shape.
—Dehydration.
—Poor posture and shallow breathing.
—Excessive stress.

Hormones, mainly estrogen, play a part in forming cellulite. Men get less cellulite deposits partly because of their naturally lower estrogen levels, and partly because of differences in their body structure. Women have more naturally-occurring fatty areas for cellulite to accumulate, such as the fat cells on their hips, thighs and buttocks which facilitate childbearing. In addition, the outer layer of a woman's skin is thinner than a man's, so the dimpled ripples of fat are more visible.

What does it take to get rid of it? Overcoming cellulite depends on re-establishing good cellular metabolism and restoring a healthy exchange between individual cells and the circulatory and lymphatic systems. Boosting circulation is one of the primary targets for achieving this goal.

Because it is unattached material, dieting and exercise alone

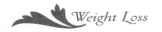

don't dislodge cellulite. Exercise can help by increasing skin and muscle tone appearance. Yet, even though weight loss diets don't work, a cleansing diet that changes body chemistry and the way the liver metabolizes fats does.

A program for cellulite release should be in four parts:
   1) It should stimulate the body's elimination functions.
   2) It should increase circulation and metabolism.
   3) It should control excess fluid retention.
   4) It should re-establish connective tissue elasticity.

Can herbal remedies help get rid of cellulite?
Herbs are good choices for improving cellulitic tissue tone, because they work at the cause of the problem, on body chemistry and metabolism, as well as on the external effect.

Your skin is a very complex organ. Regeneration of toned, elastic skin tissue works from the inside out. Man-made chemicals are often rejected by the body's system functions, but plant-derived substances can pass through the powerful metabolic defenses of the skin's upper layers.

Bioflavonoids, part of the vitamin C complex, play a key role in new collagen production, and have toning action for skin elasticity. Over 300 different types of natural flavonoids have been identified. Herbs, like *cranberries, hawthorn, bilberry and rose hips,* are an excellent source for many of them.
Herbal sources of bioflavonoids and vitamin C help preserve vein and capillary integrity, encourage new collagen formation, and make it more difficult for cellulite to begin. An herbal tea for cellulite release can easily work through the body's enzyme system to increase elimination, so that cellulitic wastes

are flushed from the body more rapidly. I recommend a high bioflavonoid herbal tea like Crystal Star's CEL-LEAN RELEASE™ tea.

Spas have been helping people reduce cellulite for hundreds of years. Today, you can use some of their effective methods in your home to help yourself.

I briefly worked in Europe at two spas during the early nineteen sixties. That experience was invaluable for learning exactly what worked and *how* it worked.

In Europe, you don't have to be wealthy, or of the "leisure class" to enjoy a spa experience. Many people take a week or two at a spa as part of their normal vacation time. They go to rejuvenate their spirits as well as their bodies, and the programs offered are far more complete than those in America, except for the most exclusive spas.

Almost every treatment that I observed was accompanied by a detoxification program and a diet regimen. Since many of the spas are in the mountains, forests or by the sea, exercise was all scheduled for outdoors, in the form of hikes, swims and games to take advantage of the incredible natural setting. Neither of the spas I lived in had workout equipment or weight rooms. There were large, quiet reading rooms for spiritual and meditation renewal.

I helped in the kitchens, so I know the food was meticulously prepared for each guest. Even in the sixties, fat was trimmed from meats, and rigorously strained from sauces and soups. Much of the fresh food was grown on the premises. Whole grain breads were baked there, too. Only goat's milk was used — from goats nearby.

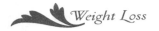

I also worked in the huge bath houses where the spa treatments were performed, so I was able to see results for myself.

Herbal body wraps help in cellulite release and improve muscle, vein and skin tone. An herbal wrap is a beauty treatment that diminishes the spongy look of cellulite tissue, by helping to squeeze it back into the working areas of the body so it can be eliminated. An accompanying detoxification program and optimally working elimination system usually guarantee the best results from a wrap. Skin improvements are often remarkably visible.

Body wraps are an inch loss, not a pound or water weight loss technique. The applied herbal extracts work by slightly changing body chemistry to increase circulation and speed up metabolism. A tight wrap streamlines the appearance of body contours, and smooths the skin. The tissue toning, internal activity of a wrap makes connective tissue less likely to re-trap the hardened waste and excess fluid that cause cellulite.

Daily self-massage after a wrap with a stimulating body lotion like Crystal Star's THERMO CEL-LEAN™ TONING GEL (This toning gel may also be applied to the skin before the body is wrapped.)

What about seaweed treatments? Does this traditional spa technique really work to reduce of cellulite?

Seaweeds add amazing luster to the skin. Eating sea vegetables or bathing in them clearly helps reduce the look of cellulite. A seaweed bath or wrap aids thyroid function, increases circulation and metabolism, and helps eliminate congestive waste through the pores. Many women report smoother skin tone and less cellulite after a seaweed treatment.

Take a seaweed bath to help reduce cellulite:

If an ocean near you has unpolluted waters, you can collect your own seaweeds (any kind works). Gather kelp and seaweeds from the water, (not the shoreline), in clean buckets or trash cans, and carry them home to your tub. If you don't live near the ocean, dried sea vegetables are available in most health food stores. Crystal Star packages a dried blend of seaweeds, gathered from the San Juan Islands, in a HOT SEAWEED BATH™.

Whichever form you choose, run very hot water over the seaweed in a tub, filling it to the point that you will be covered when you recline. The leaves will turn a beautiful bright green. The water will turn rich brown as the plants release their minerals. Add an aromatherapy bath oil if desired, to help hold the heat in and pleasantly scent the water. Let the bath cool enough to get in. As you soak, the gel from the seaweed will transfer onto your skin. This coating increases perspiration to release toxins from your system, and replaces them by osmosis with minerals. Rub your skin (especially cellulitic areas) with the sea leaves during the bath to stimulate circulation, smooth and tone the body, and remove wastes coming out on the skin surface. When the sea greens have done their therapeutic work, the gel coating dissolves and floats off the skin, and the leaves shrivel - a sign that the bath is over. Each bath varies with the individual, the seaweeds used, and water temperature, but the gel coating release is a natural timekeeper for the bath's benefits. Forty-five minutes is usually long enough to balance the acid/alkaline system, encourage liver activity, cellulite release and fat metabolism. Skin tone, color, and circulatory strength are almost immediately noticeable from iodine and potassium absorption.

Note: After the bath, take a capsule of cayenne and ginger to put these minerals quickly through the system.

To get the most from a seaweed treatment, dry brush cellulitic skin *before* your seaweed bath or wrap. This technique exfoliates dead skin, opens up the pores for improved elimination and increases circulation to the affected area.

Are thigh creams a modern miracle or modern marketing?

Theophylline, aminophylline, caffeine and theine all come from the xanthine family of stimulants. Xanthines are found in many herbs like *ephedra, kola nut* and *sida cordifolia*, and are the primary ingredient in today's popular spot reducing thigh creams. Aminophylline, a constituent of *ephedra*, is the most commercially used of the topically effective xanthines. Natural cellulite creams stimulate circulation, encourage natural elimination of cellulite wastes, and improve skin elasticity in cellulitic build up areas.

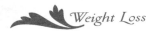

Here's how topical xanthines like theophylline and aminophylline work.

Fat cells are covered with little switches called beta-receptors. When the body needs energy, beta-receptors are stimulated to release a substance that activates fat for fuel, and then are neutralized.

The type of cells for long term fat storage, that reside in a woman's thighs and upper arms, and on a man's belly, have only a few beta-receptors and consequently hang on to their fat stores. Prolonging fat burning activity in these cells can result in one to two inches of fat loss from fat storage depots. Aminophylline's role in this process is to keep the fat releasing substance activated to prolong the fat loss mechanism.

Not all body contouring creams work the same. I've reviewed many without success. But some do work. In my experience, the best ones to reduce the look of cellulite for women are Zia Wesley-Hosford's Company Z's SLEEK & CHIC cellulite contouring cream and Chae's BODY THERAPY CONTOUR CONCENTRATE. Men seem to benefit most from Company Z's LEAN & MEAN abdominal contouring cream.

Mud pack contouring creams are another "new" old treatment for cellulite. Do they work? In ancient times, herbs and highly mineralized mud packs were used to alleviate skin problems and cellulite build-up. The best modern results we found came from CELLU-LYTE CREAM by Nature's Path - a combination of a true mineral electrolyte solution and herbs to specifically aid the breakdown of toxins within cellulite tissue.

For best results with contour packs:
• Massage and knead the contouring cream twice daily into problem areas to help break up and release cellulite deposits.
• Drink 6 - 8 glasses of water daily to flush congested wastes.
• You should see improvement in 2 months. Cellulite that used to be visible when you lay down may no longer be there.

Use an enzyme-rich diet as a key to getting rid of cellulite.
• Eat plenty of fruits and juices with vitamin C, to re-establish connective tissue elasticity and to keep the system flushed and free flowing. Citrus fruits like pineapples, are also rich in the enzyme bromelain which helps the liver metabolize fats.
• Eat chlorophyll-rich foods like leafy greens and sea vegetables to boost enzyme activity and waste elimination.
• Have Omega-rich fish and seafood twice a week.
• Graze - eat smaller, more frequent meals that are easier for your body to process instead of 2 to 3 large ones.

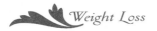

Here's the diet blacklist.
Avoid these foods to avoid cellulite.
- All fried and fatty foods
- Caffeinated drinks, carbonated drinks and hard liquor
- Red meats
- Full-fat, pasteurized dairy foods
- Salty foods - use herb seasonings and sea veggies instead

No cellulite program will work for long without liver support. Cellulitic fat is also a result of a partially exhausted or poorly functioning liver. Just as one gets "floaters" 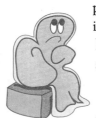 in the eyes, and brown spots on the skin when the liver is not processing wastes properly, many fats are also unmetabolized by a weak liver. Liver support herbs can help process fats through the system more normally, instead of being thrown off or stored as fatty "cottage cheese."

Herbs can tonify and regulate liver activity.
- Try a liver rebuilding herbal tonic: Mix 4-oz. hawthorn berries, 2-oz. red sage, 1-oz. cardamon. Steep for 24 hours in 2 qts. of water. Add honey. Take 2 cups daily. Add 2 teasp. royal jelly for B vitamins to assist with liver detoxification.
- Or take a liver cleansing tea, like Crystal Star LIV-ALIVE™ tea, or LIVER SUPPORT by Nature's Apothecary, especially when you take your daily enzyme therapy.
- Crystal Star CEL-LEAN™ caps help rejuvenate the liver so that it can properly metabolize fats.
- Add a carrot/beet/cucumber juice at least twice a week to clean out your liver. I have worked with this juice for years. It can literally start dumping toxins from your liver in about 30 minutes, especially when it's freshly juiced and organic.

Weight Control For Kids

Today's children are becoming an overweight generation. Until the nineteen sixties, weight control wasn't much of a problem for kids. But the fifties ushered in the fast food era - refined, chemicalized foods that changed parents' metabolism and cell structure. These parents of the fifties and sixties passed on their immune defense depletions and digestion problems to the kids of today. And that was only the beginning of the wide array of junk and chemical-laced foods and T.V. food advertising that the kids themselves are constantly exposed to.

Adults may be paying more attention to diet, but statistics show that children and teenagers are the fattest they've ever been. Too much fat, salt, sugar and calories, and too little exercise are at the root childhood weight problems. An estimated 14% of children over the age of 6 are obese - double the rate of the late 70's. Even further, U.S. schools have dropped the ball for children's health, offering kids more fatty, nutrient - starved meals and less physical exercise. P.E. classes, most sports and many extra-curricular activities have been dropped in U.S. schools and our kids are paying the price. Since 1977, $^3/_4$ of U.S. schools have either fired their P.E. teachers or reassigned them to other classes.

Today, most kids attend only 1 or 2 physical education classes a week. *Forty percent* of boys 6-12 can't touch their toes; American girls actually run slower today than they did 10 years ago (contrary to the rising standard of athletes). The telecommunications age has brought kids computers, T.V.'s, video games - all technological advances that mean less active playtime.

In the 90's, most kids watch up to 24 hours of TV a week. By the time U.S. kids reach their senior high school year, they've spent an average of 3 years of their lives watching TV.

Even more alarming, heart disease is now traceable to early childhood. U.S. doctors are discovering that many 3 year olds and teenage Americans already have fatty deposits on their coronary arteries.

Single parents, and parents holding down 2 or 3 jobs, know how difficult it is to maintain a sound, nutritious diet for kids. Today's kids rely on junk foods and many tend to overeat. **Some kids eat out of a box most of the time!**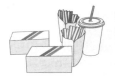

Children are rewarded with food for good behavior or denied food for punishment from an early age. As they grow older, they often continue that cycle by rewarding themselves with salty, sugary, fatty snacks, soft drinks, and nitrate-loaded lunch meats before parents even come home from work.

Add that to sedentary lifestyle, and you've got problem that could result in disaster for health. Emotional problems, family crisis or alienation from childhood peers also contribute to childhood overeating.

Overweight children face many problems including medical diseases, low self-esteem, depression and rejection by peers.

I know because I was an overweight teenager. Ice cream was my downfall. We weren't allowed to have it at home, so I ate it every chance I got. By the time I got to college, I hardly ever went to the dormitory dining room. Ice cream was practically all I ate!

Getting weight problems under control at an early age is the best choice for later health. The older an obese child is doubles the likelihood of adult obesity. But, crash diets are not the solution for kids (or adults.) Changing the focus to health, to having a fit body instead of a thin body can make all the difference in a weight management program for everybody.

Snacks, lunch foods and meals can be satisfying and delicious without adding significant amounts of sugar, fat or salt. Kids need mineral-rich building foods, fiber-rich energy foods, and protein-rich growth foods. Since metabolism and energy are naturally high in most kids, changing the type of food eaten is easy and spontaneous.

Here are some weight loss tips you can use for childhood weight control problems. I usually recommend a light detox to start. A child's body often has "toxic overload" from too many chemical-laced foods. A very gentle detox normalizes body chemistry before beginning a healthy diet program.

My JUNK FOOD DETOX FOR KIDS is a 3 day diet. Avoid all highly processed junk foods, red meats and dairy products, except for yogurt during this detox.

On rising: give citrus juice with 1 teaspoon of acidophilus liquid, or $^1/_4$ teasp. acidophilus powder; or a glass of lemon juice and water with honey or maple syrup.

Breakfast: offer fresh fruits, such as apples, pineapple, papaya or oranges. Add vanilla yogurt or soymilk if desired.

Mid-morning: Give fresh carrot juice. Add $^1/_4$ teasp. ascorbate vitamin C or Ester C crystals to neutralize body toxins.

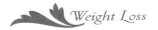

Lunch: give fresh raw crunchy veggies with a yogurt dip; or a fresh veggie salad with lemon/oil or yogurt dressing.

Mid-afternoon: offer a refreshing herb tea, such as licorice or peppermint tea with honey.

Dinner: give a fresh salad, with avocados, carrots, kiwi, romaine and other high vitamin A foods; and/or a cup of miso soup or other clear broth soup.

Before bed: offer a relaxing herb tea, like chamomile tea, or Crystal Star GOOD NIGHT TEA™. Add $1/4$ teasp. ascorbate vitamin C or Ester C crystals; or a cup of MISO broth for strength and B vitamins.

Note: I recommend herbal baths, washes and compresses to neutralize and cleanse toxins coming out through the skin during the cleanse. Give a soothing massage before bed. Give your child an early morning sunbath or playtime every day possible for regenerating vitamin D.

Once your child's light detox is over, use it as a fresh start for a healthy diet. Breakfast is a key for weight loss for kids. Both kids and adults who eat a high fiber breakfast don't feel as hungry at lunchtime, and eat an average of 200 fewer calories during the day.

Here are some weight control diet tips for kids:

Incorporate plenty of fresh, enzyme-rich foods in the child's diet. Enzymes are critical to healthy digestion. Many of today's diet don't work because they rely on microwaved foods - a process that kills the enzymes. Overcooked foods, microwaved foods and junk foods are all enzyme deficient.

There is no question that our modern diet of devitalized, "enzyme dead" foods is creating a nutritional gap for our kids.

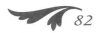

For some children, this also means weight gain and constipation, a major problem for kids that eat a lot of dairy foods like milk, cheese and ice cream and red meats. 20% of Caucasian children and 80% of black children don't produce lactase, the enzyme necessary to digest milk.

Here are two enzyme rich juice recipes that even the pickiest of kids will ask for again and again.

#1 GREEN DRINK FOR KIDS

Make it in a juicer. Make it easy. Use any fresh veggies that your child likes most. Be sure to include some green leafy vegetables like spinach, sunflower greens and lettuces.

I find that kids like baby veggies. Consider baby bok choy, baby carrots and sprouts. Don't forget sweet tasting veggies like cucumbers, celery and tomatoes.

#2 ENERGIZING FRUIT SMOOTHIE

Always use fresh fruit (organic if possible), for this drink, not canned or frozen. Blend 1 BANANA and 1 ORANGE with apple juice. Add half a papaya or mango if available, or one-quarter of a fresh pineapple.

If you don't have a juicer, at the very least, give your child a good plant enzyme supplement to keep his system free and flowing, and metabolism going strong. Plant enzymes can help get a child over the "hump" of a weight problem. Even highly sensitive children with food allergies can tolerate high quality plant enzymes. Digestive plant enzymes help kids break down foods to ensure optimum digestion and absorption of nutrients, and also can relieve digestive symptoms like constipation, gas, bloat, and diarrhea.

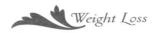

I recommend a mealtime supplement with plant enzymes like Prevail's CHILDREN'S DIGESTION FORMULA, or Transformation's POWDERED DIGEST ZYME, both quality products that I've worked with.

The following diet serves as an easy weight control guideline for kids. It has passed many tests on both overweight and "couch potato" kids for foods that they will eat. It focuses on nutrition, so your child will have LESS CRAVING for junk foods that may cause him or her to put on weight.

On rising: give a vitamin/mineral drink such as NutriTech EARTHSHAKE or Nature's Plus SPIRU-TEIN (lots of flavors), or 1 tsp. liquid multi-vitamin in juice (such as Floradix CHILDREN'S MULTI-VITAMIN/MINERAL).

Breakfast: have a whole grain cereal with apple juice or a little yogurt and fresh fruit;

If more is desired, add whole grain toast or muffins, with butter, kefir cheese or nut butter; add eggs, scrambled or baked or soft boiled (no fried eggs);

or have some hot oatmeal or kashi with a little maple syrup and yogurt if desired.

Mid-morning: snacks can be whole grain crackers with kefir cheese or low-fat cheese or dip, and a sugarless juice or sparkling mineral water;

and/or some fresh fruit, like apples with yogurt or kefir cheese, or fruit leather;

or fresh crunchy veggies, like celery, with peanut butter;

or a no-sugar dried fruit, nut and seed candy bar, or a dried fruit and nut trail mix, stirred into yogurt.

Lunch: have a veggie burger, or a turkey sandwich on whole grain bread, with low-fat cheese and low fat mayonnaise;

Add whole grain or corn chips with a low-fat veggie or cheese dip; or a hearty bean soup with whole grain toast or crackers, and crunchy veggies with garbanzo spread;

or a baked potato with a butter, kefir cheese, or low fat cheese, and a green salad;

or a vegetarian pizza on a chapati or whole grain crust;

or a Mexican bean and veggie, or rice or whole wheat burrito with a light, natural no-sugar salsa.

Mid-afternoon: have a sparkling juice and a dried fruit candy bar, or fruit juice-sweetened cookies;

or some fresh fruit or fruit juice, or a kefir drink with whole grain muffins and kefir cheese;

or a hard boiled egg, and some whole grain chips with a low-fat cheese dip;

or some whole grain toast and peanut butter.

Dinner: have whole grain spaghetti or pasta with a light sauce and parmesan cheese, or whole grain or egg pasta with vegetables and a light tomato/cheese sauce;

or a baked Mexican quesadilla with low-fat cheese and some steamed vegetables or a salad;

or a stir-fry with crunchy noodles, brown rice, baked egg rolls and a light soup;

or some roast turkey with corn bread dressing and a salad;

or a dinner omelet. I find most kids like omelets with steamed veggies, shrimp, or cheese and bean filling;

or a tuna casserole with rice, peas and water chestnuts and toasted chapatis with a little butter.

T.V. snack: a snack of unbuttered, spicy, savory popcorn is good and nutritious anytime.

Before bed: a glass of apple juice, rice amazake drink (from your health food store) or vanilla soy milk or flavored kefir.

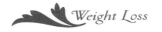
Here are some other diet tips to help keep your child healthier and happier:

I know it's a lot easier said than done to change old dietary patterns to more healthful eating....for anybody, but especially for kids. A good way to start is to offer something delicious to replace whatever is being taken away.

For example:

• If you want to include more wholesome foods, like fruits and vegetables, start with food forms that children naturally go for - like dried fruit snacks, and smoothies for fruits. Sandwiches, tacos, burritos and pitas can hold vegetables. Most kids like soup.... another good place to add vegetables. Let them add sauces or flavors they like.

• If you want to include more whole grains in a child's diet, start by keeping only whole grains in the house. Kids love bagels, and there are lots of healthy choices. Pastas come in a wide variety of whole grain options. Brown or basmati rice is much tastier than white rice if your kid is a " rice kid." Stuffing is already a big favorite with kids - make sure it's whole grain. Popcorn is a healthy snack. (Season it with tamari or a healthy season blend rather than gobs of butter and salt.)

• If you want to add healthy cultured foods to your child's diet, start by keeping a good assortment of yogurt flavors with fruit for snacks in the fridge. Offer delicious kefir cheese for snack spreads instead of sour cream.

• If you want to reduce the amount of sugar your child is consuming, your health food store has a wide variety of delicious, sugar-free snacks. Replace sugar-filled cereals with granolas

and oatmeal with toppings. Offer dried fruit, too. Almost every kid likes raisins.

• If you want to reduce the amount of meat and heavy dairy proteins your child is eating, keep good plant protein available. Kids like tofu and grain burgers, especially with their favorite trimmings. Most kids like beans, too - look for healthy chili blends. Keep peanut butter, and nuts and seeds, like almonds, sunflower seeds and pumpkin seeds around the house for snacks; recommend them as toppings for everything from soup or salad crunchies to smoothies and desserts. (Seeds and nuts give kids unsaturated oils and essential fatty acids, too.)

Eggs are a good protein choice for kids...one of Nature's perfect foods that's gotten a bad rap. Most kids like deviled eggs, and eggs are great in honey custards, another kid favorite.

• If you want to add more fish and seafood to a child's diet, start with a favorite like shrimp, tuna fish or salmon.

• If you want to encourage your child to drink more water, instead of carbonated sodas or sweet drinks, keep plenty of natural fruit juices and flavored mineral water around the house.

Exercise is the key to health, weight management, growth and body oxygen. No weight loss program for kids will work without it. Don't let your kid be a couch potato, or a computer junkie. Encourage outdoor sports and activity every day possible, and make sure he or she is taking P. E. classes at school. Exercise for kids is one of the best nutrients for both body and mind.

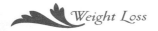
Eating Disorders

What about eating disorders? Some weight loss programs are so severe that following them blindly can be dangerous and put you on a fine line between health and self-destruction. For over thirty-five percent of American women and over seventy-five percent of American teen-age girls, looking good means being bone thin. American females are told from an early age that "fat" is bad.

Young women and teenage girls are especially affected. The newest studies indicate that as early as the fifth and sixth grade, almost 70% of girls have tried to lose weight but only a third of them needed to. One out of a hundred young women between ages 10 to 20 are starving themselves. One in 4 college women has bulimia.

Fashion models are presented as both the aesthetic standard *and the health standard.* Striving to meet this abnormal standard translates to thinness at any cost - specifically to eating disorders that are extremely hard to overcome, and which eventually result in disabling health problems.

Within 20 years of an eating disorder diagnosis, there is a mortality rate of almost 40%! Men are not completely exempt. Bodybuilders, male models, etc. have competition from ever-thinner rivals, and can suffer low testicular function from starving. Today, men comprise 10% of people with eating disorders.

Have you dieted to the point where you have lost the desire to eat? Eating disorders throw your body so completely out of balance that it can't "talk" to you. Normal food cravings that your body uses as signals to tell you that it needs certain nutrients to keep you healthy are no longer active.

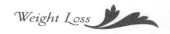

Do you have an eating disorder?

Take the test on this page. If you are concerned about yourself or someone else, the following questions can help you determine whether there might be a problem.

If you answer yes to one or more of the questions, you may be suffering from an eating disorder. Getting help is essential to recovery. Eating disorders are progressive and can result in death.

- Do you always feel fat?
- Have you repeatedly tried and failed to lose weight?
- Do you ever fast or put yourself on incredibly strict diets?
- Are you preoccupied with food?
- Do you hide your eating habits from others?
- Is there a relationship between your eating and your self-esteem? Do you feel you have lost control?
- Do you sometimes binge, or eat large amounts of food in a short period of time?
- Have you ever tried to "undo" the damage of eating by vomiting, taking laxatives or fasting?
- Do you exercise compulsively? Do you feel guilty or fat if you miss your regular exercise schedule?
- Do you eat when you are under stress or depressed?
- Are you a vegetarian solely to be thin, or is it for other reasons?
- Do you feel guilty when you eat meat and dairy, or caloric and high-fat vegetarian foods?
- Do you prepare food for others but refuse to eat it yourself? Do you stick to a rigid routine of eating?
- Do you still think you're fat even after losing a substantial amount of weight?
- How do your weight loss goals compare with what weight charts suggest for someone of your height?

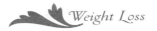

What are eating disorders exactly? If you took the test on the last page and feel you may be at risk, check out the following descriptions to see which eating disorder pattern is affecting you.

Bulimia is characterized by a secretive cycle of binge eating then purging the body with laxatives, diuretics, vomiting or compulsive exercise. Surveys indicate that almost ten percent of U.S. women suffer from bulimia at some point in their lives. Symptoms include a swollen neck and eroded tooth enamel from excessive vomiting, broken blood vessels on the face, low pulse rate and blood pressure, and extreme weakness. Bulimics are frequently severely dehydrated and malnourished. Some may actually rupture their esophagus from compulsive vomiting.

Anorexia is characterized by a refusal to eat, preoccupation with feeling fat and an obsession with food. Anorexia is diagnosed when a woman is already 15% below normal weight and has not menstruated in three months. Anorexics sometimes cook for others while denying themselves meals. The physical toll of anorexia is enormous. Symptoms include reduced metabolism, cold hands and feet, dry skin, brittle, dull hair, tooth decay and yellow teeth, chronic constipation and cessation of menses. Body temperature, heart rate, and blood pressure become dangerously low with anorexia. There is risk of cardiac failure from loss of potassium and severe malnutrition. Some women suffer from anorexia and bulimia at the same time.

Binge-eating disorder is a syndrome marked by an out-of-control compulsion to eat abnormally large amounts of food in a short period of time. A binge eater consumes lots of food much faster than normal, to the point of feeling uncomfortably full and bloated. As many as $1/4$ of young women go on food binging cycles that interfere with their lives. Binge-eating can cause weight gain and obesity, leading to a score of health problems like diabetes, hypertension, circulatory problems, hormonal imbalances and cardiovascular disease.

Eating disorders are usually caused by complex cultural or emotional problems that end up turning into a form of compulsive psychosis. A traumatic event, a long period of chronic stress or emotional pain, or a mood disorder such as depression can trigger an eating disorder. Some studies link low levels of serotonin and norepinephrine in the brain to eating disorders.

Seeking help for emotional factors linked to eating disorders is important for long term recovery. Since there is a high correlation between sexual abuse and eating disorders, psychological counseling is often helpful.

It can help in understanding the almost universal problem of low self-esteem that triggers this type of harmful behavior, and in effectively dealing with it. Therapy during healing reinforces the idea that destructive thinking and behavior can change, and self-confidence of the patient re-established.

Can natural therapies help when dieting goes too far? Stabilizing the body with natural therapies while changing lifestyle habits helps overcome eating disorders. Here are some tips to replenish lost nutrients, rebuild body strength, and restore nervous system health to jumpstart healing.

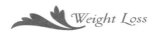
First: Change your diet habits.

• Eat a high vegetable protein, complex carbohydrate diet. Always eat breakfast, with whole grain cereals, especially cooked grains(like brown rice or oatmeal), fruit, yogurt, etc.

• Don't skip meals.

• Avoid all junk foods, especially heavy starches like white flour pastries, buns, doughnuts and gluey turnovers, and sugary foods like cakes and ice creams. They disrupt normalization of body chemistry.

• Eat slowly and chew well. Have small meals often for best absorption.

• Make a mix of toasted wheat germ, blackstrap molasses and brewer's yeast, (or a yeast product like Red Star NUTRITIONAL YEAST MINI FLAKES). Take 2TBS. daily of the mix for dietary B vitamins.

— Or consider TOTAL-LYTE by Nature's Path. It has a unique yeast formula with exceptionally broad-scoped, highly absorbable complete protein, with amino acids, RNA/DNA for cell development, vitamins, and minerals.

Second: Superfoods can be lifesavers. Here are some superfoods I have found helpful for eating disorders.

• Crystal Star SYSTEMS STRENGTH™ formula rebuilds foundation strength.

• Have a daily protein drink like Nappi THE PERFECT MEAL or Solgar WHEY TO GO. Crystal Star nutrient-rich LIGHT WEIGHT HERBAL DIET PLAN™ drink is well-accepted by people struggling with eating disorders. It has satisfying nutrition requirements without excess calories or any fats.

• Carrot juice daily or Green Foods BETA CARROT.

• Y.S. ROYAL JELLY 3-4 teasp. daily for B vitamins and to rebuild adrenal health. (Eating disorders exhaust the adrenals.)

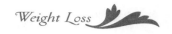

Third: Mineral therapy is effective.

• A load of minerals are lost from vomiting and laxatives. Girls don't realize that the very minerals they lose through vomiting are the ones that help them control their weight. Potassium and iodine stimulate the thyroid to keep metabolism, and therefore calorie-burning, strong. Minerals also help to regain normal menstrual periods.

Adding sea vegetables as a salad, soup or vegetarian pizza sprinkle are my favorite choice. You get a load of the very minerals you need in a very small quantity of food. (They're full of bioflavonoids and fatty acids for tissue, collagen production, capillary strength and skin tone, too.)

• Zinc is a key mineral for eating disorder healing. Severely zinc-deficient people can't manufacture a key protein that allows them to taste, and they tend to lose even more desire for food.

• Anorexia is associated with weak, brittle bones, nails and hair, and peeling skin. These conditions often dramatically improve with silicon supplementation. I have worked with BIOSIL by Jarrow Formulas and SILICA SOURCE™ drops by Crystal Star with good results.

• Eating disorders severely deplete calcium stores in the body, reducing the tone and elasticity of muscles and ligaments. (This is one of the reasons late-stage anorexics and bulimics become too weak to stand or walk.) Calcium from herbs is better processed and more easily bioavailable than calcium from pasteurized dairy products. I recommend CALCIUM SOURCE™ by Crystal Star or CALCIUM & MAGNESIUM by Solaray (amino acid chelates in a base of mineral-rich herbs.)

• Here are some mineral products for eating disorders. Crystal Star POTASSIUM/IODINE SOURCE™ caps to replenish lost minerals and nourish the thyroid, Mezotrace SEA MINERAL COMPLEX, and Nature's Path TRACE-LYTE (liquid crystalloid mineral electrolytes). Electrolytes are essential for the existence of life (you lose them along with minerals during vomiting). They help your body maintain proper blood pressure, use the nutrients you give it, rebuild damaged tissues, expedite waste from the body and balance your body's pH.

Fourth: Use herbs to stimulate appetite and digestion.

• GINSENG/GOTU KOLA caps act as a tonic adaptogen to restore appetite and energy.

• Take an acidophilus complex powder, $^1/_4$ teasp. 3x daily in water for "friendly bacteria" with a high quality, plant enzyme supplement for absorption like Rainbow Light's ADVANCED ENZYME SYSTEM.

• REZYME by Nature's Secret

• DIGESTZYME by Transformation Enzyme.

Fifth: Reduce stress.

• A GABA compound for stress relief and nerve health like GABA-PLUS by Twinlab.

• Crystal Star's RELAX CAPS™ 2 daily to rebuild and normalize nerve structure.

Sixth: Develop your life support system.

• Cultivate relationships with positive people, in whose company you feel good about yourself.

• Get some mild exercise every day for lung, heart and muscle rebuilding.

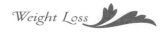

* Get regular massage therapy treatments - at least once a month for several months to relax and normalize.

Summary

Weight loss is not easy in today's lifestyle. Reaching your ideal weight is a victory. Keeping it requires vigilance in light of today's processed food products and fast lifestyles. But it can be successful on a long-term basis, and without side effects.

Here are some watchwords:

1) The four keys to an effective weight control diet are low fat, high fiber, regular exercise and plenty of water.

2) Try to lose 1% of your body weight per week. More than that and the body doesn't adjust properly. You will probably end up regaining the weight.

3) Don't worry about the pounds and the calories. Muscle is heavy. Worry about the inches and the fat.

4) Adding exercise to your life and correcting your diet composition takes inches off 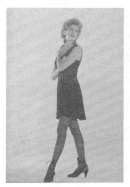 a lot faster than pounds. So forget the scale. Look at yourself in the mirror. Watch your clothing size go down! It is a real achievement!

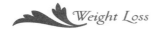

Product Resource List

The following listing is included for your convenience in obtaining the products recommended in the Healthy Healing Library Series. The list is unsolicited by the companies named. Healthy Healing is continually developing healing and wellness programs with products you can access easily and inexpensively. We initiate contact with each company and review the quality and effectiveness of specific products we plan to test and work with.

There are many other fine companies not listed here, but you can have every assurance we can offer that the products we recommend are effective and safe.

Anabol Naturals, 1550 Mansfield St., Santa Cruz, CA 95062, 408-479-1403

Body Ecology, 295 King Road, Atlanta GA 30342, 800-478-3842

Crystal Star Herbal Nutr., 6305 Wedgeway Ct., Earth City, MO, 800-736-6015

Ethical Nutrients, 971 Calle Negocio, San Clemente, CA 92673, 714-366-0818

Frontier Natural Products, P.O. Box 299, Norway, IA 52318, 800-669-3275

Futurebiotics, 72 Cotton Mill Hill, A24, Brattleboro, VT 05301, 800-367-5433

Gaia Herbs, Inc., 12 Lancaster County Road, Harvard, MA 01451, 800-831-7780

Green Foods Corp., 320 North Graves Ave., Oxnard, CA 93030 800-777-4430

Jarrow Formulas, 1824 Robertson Blvd., Los Angeles, CA 90035 800-726-0886

Maine Coast Sea Vegetables, RR1 Box 78, Franklin, Maine 04634, 207-565-2907

MRI (Medical Research Institute), 2160 Pacific, Suite 61, San Francisco CA 94115, 888-448-4246

Natural Balance, 3130 N. Commerce, Castle Rock, CO 80104, 303-688-6633

Nature's Apothecary, 6350 Gunpark Dr. #500, Boulder, CO 80301, 800-999-7422

Nature's Path, P.O. Box 7862, Venice, FL 34287, 800-326-5772

Nature's Secret, 5485 Conestoga Ct., Boulder, CO80301, 303-546-6306

Nova Homeopathics, 5600 McLeod NE. Suite F, Albuquerque, NM 87109, 800-225-8094

NutriCology, Box 489, 400 Preda Street, San Leandro, CA 94577, 800-545-9960

Source Naturals Inc. 23 Janis Way, Scotts Valley, CA 95066, 800-777-5677

Transformation Enzyme Corp., 2900 Wilcrest Suite 220, Houston, TX 77042, 800-777-1474

Wakunaga of America, 23501 Madero, Mission Viejo, CA 92691, 800-825-7888